How to Naturally Produce and Increase Testosterone Levels

By: Nick Stanton

Published by:
Nick Stanton and Random Technologies
4409 HOFFNER AVENUE, 347
Belle Isle, FL 32812
Website: www.MensGrowth.com

Disclaimer

All rights reserved. No part of this book may be reproduced or transmitted in any manner whatsoever without written permission, except in the case of brief quotations used in articles and reviews.

This book is intended as reference material and not as a medical manual to replace the advice of your physician or to substitute for any treatment prescribed by your physician.

If you are ill or suspect that you have a medical problem, we strongly encourage you to consult your medical, health or other competent professional before adopting any of the suggestions in this book or drawing inferences from it. If you are taking prescription medication, you should never change your diet (for better or worse) without consulting your physician as any dietary change may affect the metabolism of that prescription drug.

This book and the author's opinions are solely for informational and educational purposes.

The author specifically disclaims all responsibility for any liability, loss or risk, personal or otherwise which is incurred as a consequence, directly or indirectly, of the use and application of any of the contents of this book. Individual results may vary.

Thank You for Choosing our Book!

Your purchase means a lot to us, and we hope this report on Increasing Your Testosterone Naturally meets your expectations.

Sign Up for Your
FREE UNADVERTISED BONUS:
www.mensgrowth.com/join

Table of Contents

Welcome

So you're interested in enhancing your testosterone levels. Good! I have discussed this matter with groups of men over the years, and believe me, many of us could use a bit more testosterone in our lives... Testosterone benefits guys in a number of ways, some of which you may be aware and others that may come as a complete surprise.

Did you know that increased levels of testosterone are associated with:

- Creating and Maintaining a Solid Erection…
- Feelings of Youth and Virility...
- Feelings of Power and Stamina…
- Sexual Satisfaction and Passion…
- Your Health and Vitality …

Are you aware that, despite the benefits of testosterone, your body doesn't retain it very well as you age? In fact, you lose a quarter of your base testosterone level by the time you're just in your mid-fifties! There are many factors that influence your testosterone levels, ranging from alcohol intake to diet and more. Don't be afraid; you *can* fight this process!

- ✓ If you're ready to move past feeling exhausted all the time
- ✓ If you're done accepting these symptoms as "a normal part of aging"
- ✓ If you want to feel strong and confident as you once did

You're reading the right book!

This guide not only seeks to help you rebuild your levels of testosterone but to do so naturally – no little blue pills, gels, shots or surgeries necessary. We'll focus on ways to combat testosterone loss that occur as you age, we'll look at how you can to restore your energy and we'll help you understand the science behind it all. By examining the existing research and reaping the benefits, you can increase your testosterone levels -- naturally.

We also look into helping you become healthier in every aspect of your life. This guide contains tips to:

- Learn to eat in ways that benefit your masculinity and health
- Help you to lose weight and create more muscle
- Improve your focus, lift your spirits and banish depression
- Claim your birthright as a man with healthy levels of testosterone

Too many men have suffered in silence for too long. They have this vague feeling that something is missing from their everyday lives but unable to identify precisely what is lacking.

I intend to walk you through some of the lessons my discussions with other men have enabled me to learn. I owe a huge debt of gratitude to all who helped make this book a reality by inspiring my research and to the medical professionals I consulted who helped me fact-check my findings.

Congratulations and welcome to '***How to Naturally Produce and Increase Testosterone Levels***'! I hope this will be the beginning of a personal transformation for you as well as some enjoyable improvements to your life.

What is Testosterone Deficiency?

So what exactly is a testosterone deficiency? Sure, it's clearly a lack of testosterone, but what does that mean for you?

1. Everything You Need to Know About Testosterone

Testosterone is an androgen, a type of steroid hormone responsible for the production of masculine traits and behaviors. So how does testosterone affect your personal life?

- First and foremost, it is a hormone. Hormones are chemical messengers that facilitate communication between various parts of your body. Testosterone in particular sends a message of arousal and a signal to produce sperm.

- It's also a steroid. Steroids are chemicals your body naturally produces to promote cell restoration and growth. Steroids also increase muscle and bone mass.

- Testosterone is an androgen. Like estrogen and progestagen, androgen is a sex steroid. Androgen plays a role in the virilization process, or the production of masculine behaviors and characteristics.

Testosterone production occurs primarily in the testicles, with small amounts secreted by the adrenal glands (a particularly small set of endocrine glands located atop the kidneys). Interestingly, testosterone plays a role in the womb by determining gender.

All embryos initially appear female. Embryos destined to become males make the transition at approximately the sixth week of the gestation period when these soon-to-be male embryos are dosed with testosterone. Testosterone striking at this time does indeed appear to be the key factor in the shifting of embryo's gender, and these strikes continue throughout a young man's life.

We have all heard the joke about 'raging hormones' but the truth is testosterone does indeed spike at two separate points in a young boy's life -- at birth and at puberty. These spikes appear to help the body maintain its levels of testosterone as the body loses most of the embryonic hormone by the time the birthing process occurs. The second burst occurs approximately eleven years later.

Of course, the pubertal testosterone spike is one that lasts substantially longer and can cause confusion as boys become men. Between sexual urges, the drive to compete and the instinctual search for a female, testosterone can create a host of new situations for a young lad. Indeed, this hormonal spike is the beginning of his manhood.

What Does It Do?

Testosterone has three primary effects on the body: anabolism (the building of tissues in the area it affects), virilization and sexual arousal of the penis.

How Does It Work?

Testosterone is produced within two places in the body, the testes and the adrenal glands. Once formed, it is metabolized through the use of your body's enzymes supply and delivered to the areas of the body that need it.

Notably, this metabolization process can either break the hormone down into DHT (dihydrotestosterone), as in men, *or* into estradiol (a hormone found primarily in women).

When and Where Did we Discover Testosterone?

Testosterone was first recognized in 1935 through the research of a Dutch scientist who detected its presence in the testes of mice. Soon thereafter, the German biologist Adolf Butenandt created a chemical copy of testosterone.

2. Other Androgens in the Body

Did You Know That Testosterone is not the only Androgen Your Body Produces?

The body produces testosterone but it also produces other androgens called dihydrotestosterone (DHT) and dehydropiandrosterone (DHEA).

That said, DHT is a form of testosterone and DHEA becomes what is known as androstenedione when metabolized (a chemical which the body then converts into... wait for it ... testosterone).

Each of these androgens has specialized functions. DHT enables a wider distribution of testosterone and DHEA boosts your health as well as your testosterone level. The unfortunate reality is that DHT requires testosterone to exist and DHEA also leaves the body over time – leaving the male testosterone low despite androgens the body keeps in reserve.

Why is a low testosterone level problematic? The decline in male's testosterone levels is markedly linked to several negative health effects and quality of life factors. Interestingly, the lack of testosterone is linked to the rise of estrogen in the body. Both occur naturally and are caused by environmental influences.

For example, did you know that estrogen is often added to our food? Estrogen helps livestock to gain weight rapidly, thus increasing their market value when slaughtered. But what happens when that steak or pork chop is delivered to your table? <u>You're ingesting doses of a hormone that causes feminization in males!</u>

Some men reluctantly vow to give up red meat for the sake of remaining virile but it wouldn't help. The truth is, sources of the highest levels of estrogen are actually fowl (chickens and turkeys specifically) and animal by-products such as eggs and dairy. Apparently, estrogen can't be avoided in one's diet. Fret not, dear reader -- we can help!

3. Aging and Testosterone

If the spikes of testosterone that occur at birth and during puberty lasted forever, testosterone would remain stable throughout a man's life. But the research on this subject is clear -- a man's level of testosterone consistently declines over time.

In fact, Dr. Fernand Labrie and his colleagues at the Canadian University Center Hospital recently published a study indicating this testosterone decline could begin as early as age 25! Follow-up research done by the New York Academy of Sciences found that from the age of 25 - 35 you have already lost 25% of the androgens in your body! The fact that these declines continue throughout life leaves the average man with a mere 27% - 43% of his original testosterone levels by the time he's reached the age of 80.

I'm sure you've already heard about aging and your body. Your metabolism slows down and your need for sleep increases yet your ability to fulfill it decreases. Your abdominal six pack that was once a source of pride now looks more like a pot belly. The truth is, as bad as some of these changes sound, these are just the physical manifestations of aging.

For women, this is the time of life when menopause kicks in. Thank goodness us men don't have to worry about that, right? Not so fast, years of research by Jonathon V. Wright, M.D. and his colleague Lane Leonard, Ph.D. indicates there is a similar pattern within males called “andropause.”

So what are the symptoms of this condition that awaits you?

- Problems sleeping

- Persistent fatigue: That sudden “need to take a nap” that you've never experienced before, and the little amount of sleep you are able to obtain doesn't seem to help.

- Inability to obtain or maintain an erection: Long gone are the days when you could pop up when you're ready and stay there until you're 'done.' This symptom can be particularly damaging to one's sense of manhood.

- Premature or absent ejaculations: These manifestations include having difficulty achieving orgasm, achieving orgasm too quickly (yikes) or being completely unable to achieve orgasm at all.

- Reduced overall sex drive: Finding yourself faking it more? Lacking that lusty passion you and your wife once had? This could be symptomatic of a bigger problem with aging.

- Muscle mass decline: It's not your imagination; your arms really are getting smaller! Statistically speaking, on average a man will lose three pounds of muscular mass every ten years.

- Depression and irritability: These problems are often associated with a lack of sleep but they impact far more than your night life. Being cranky and unmotivated can be a huge drain on not just you but on your loved ones. If you don't seek treatment for these issues you run the risk of permanent relationship damage.

- Osteoporosis: This disease affects 20% of men across the world.

- Thinning skin: From the length of time to recover from a cut or stress on your body to how easily you bruise -- these are all consequences of thinning skin. How much different your skin is from when you were younger!

- Increased risk of heart disease and prostate cancer

- Issues maintaining focus

- Memory blanks: Nobody likes a faulty memory, as it reminds us we're getting older. However, it is also a symptom of andropause!

Sounds fun, doesn't it? When broken down etymologically, the word andropause literally means "the completion of manhood." Much like menopause, it not only drains men physically, but emotionally. So it's not just women who have these life changes.

Many of these symptoms have mistakenly been identified thus far only in women. Hence, menopause has long been on the medical radar of health professionals. Dr. Wright cautions against ignoring the effects of andropause, suggesting that his research indicates men experience significant declines in testosterone, just as women experience declines in progesterone and estrogen. What do these hormones have in common? They are each linked to their prospective sexes.

The male rate of age-related testosterone loss (remember that distinction; age is not the only way we lose testosterone) is about 1% loss per year.

3. The Decline of Testosterone – Is It Just Natural?

So we've established that men's testosterone levels decline as they age. Moreover, thanks to environmental reasons, today they also have rising estrogen levels. The fact that so many men experience this decline often gives the illusion of normalcy. Thus, many people believe the myth that this decline is "natural."

Although there are certain natural changes to the body that can affect hormone levels, the loss of testosterone and increase in estrogen has also been linked to the use of chemicals, pesticides and even adulterants present in our food. Our environment plays a large part in explaining the extreme loss of testosterone in men.

4. The Good News?

You may not be able to prevent yourself from aging but you do have control over your environment. Testosterone loss can be prevented and even reversed to a certain degree.

You can begin the process of reversal when you're in your 40s as you experience these changes. Prevention can even start when you're in your 20s -- when you should be standing up for your right to remain a man.

5. How Testosterone Deficiency Affects You

The best known effect of a testosterone deficiency is decreased sex drive and desire. This can manifest itself by difficulty in maintaining an erection, shrinkage of the penis and decreased sperm count. But this is far from the only effect a lack of testosterone produces within your body. Much research has studied the effects of testosterone; this chapter reviews some of the literature.

The Study

In 2008 the 'Journal of Social Psychology' published a study investigating the effects of testosterone. They found that testosterone was actually linked to societal status. The study was focused on competition, who won or lost (creating a status situation) and why.

To study the effects of competition on the body's hormone secretion, the first experiment was performed with an all-male sample. The experiment revealed that men who had high levels of testosterone and lost the competition had significantly elevated levels of cortisol (a well-known stress hormone). On the other hand, those men who had high levels of testosterone and won had significantly lower levels of cortisol (a seemingly apt reward for winning). Interestingly, men with lower base levels of testosterone did not have any significant cortisol interactions despite the outcome of the competition. Hence testosterone is isolated as the key factor in this sample.

The following experiment compared cortisol results of men with the results of competition on women's cortisol levels. Similar effects were found. Women high in testosterone who won were less stressed, and indeed wanted to repeat the experiment, whereas women with lower levels of testosterone who lost were stressed and wanted to go no further with the competition. Once again, those lower in testosterone levels did not show differential preferences, again implicating testosterone as the identifying factor.

The researchers concluded that people with higher levels of testosterone have extra motivation to seek status (in this case, winning) because of the cortisol effect – a condition not present in their counterparts with lower testosterone levels!

The Follow Ups

The psychology department at Wayne State University in Detroit published a follow up study in 2011 which correlated levels of testosterone with success in vying for the affections of an attractive woman and social dominance.

Their study showed that the most successful groups were both high in testosterone and reported a need for social dominance; they were rewarded by achieving that goal.

So...

While you may have been aware before that testosterone was related to your sex life (we'll talk about that more later), I bet you weren't aware it was also related to your social status and competitive success!

This conclusion isn't just from a psychology laboratory experiment. The most successful tennis players tend to have more testosterone than their inferior counterparts, and lawyers and businessmen have more testosterone than their less corporate counterparts.

Think about what this means as you age and progressively lose more and more testosterone. People high in testosterone tend to come out winners in life. What does this mean for you?

A lack of testosterone is not just linked to a reduction in sexual desire but also to low self-esteem, a lack of drive for status and stamina issues. Your body loses muscle and struggles to hold posture correctly. Your body even recovers from cuts differently when your levels of testosterone are lower.

The Testosterone Solution – How to Stop Decline and Reverse Damage

So if the goal is to have high testosterone, and you have diminished levels already in your body, what do you think you need to do? The answer may seem simple, and it is -- you need to regain the lost testosterone and slow the ongoing decline!

Now, while the answer is simple, it's not quite so simple to do. It's not as though you can drink testosterone-inducing juice, or take a pill every morning to keep yourself up in androgens. (In fact, you cannot ingest testosterone without seriously damaging your liver.) Ask any athlete who has tried to supplement *his* levels with a little steroid boosting. It just doesn't work – it will hurt your body more than it helps. In fact, there are a lot of ineffective ways to boost your testosterone levels however temporary their effects may be.

1. What Shouldn't You Do?

You could seek medical attention, thinking that perhaps a prescription might help. Think again. Consider the following before seeking medical outcomes.

Testosterone must be taken via injection to be properly accepted into your bloodstream. You might think a little pain from a small hypodermic is a worthy tradeoff for testosterone. But testosterone is a thick substance – akin to 50 weight motor oil – and I think you will find that the needle is not so small, nor the pain so slight, when testosterone is injected. Once you realize that a regular regimen of testosterone injections is needed for any noticeable difference you are likely to reconsider this option.

The level of pain you experience from injecting testosterone should serve as a sufficient deterrent but medical attention also has other negative impacts. A prescription for testosterone can be costly and often requires careful medical supervision when taken. Beyond all these practical concerns, injecting testosterone into your body has serious consequences.

Testosterone produced naturally does not harm the body but testosterone injections and prescriptions have been associated with water retention, liver and prostate damage, rapid weight gain and high blood pressure. All are highly undesirable side effects and can be completely avoided.

By now you no doubt realize if the use of synthetic testosterone is problematic then natural forms of testosterone are a preferable solution. Here's the great news – doctors have conducted research into utilizing safe and natural ways to boost testosterone effectively and found a number of effective treatment options.

2. The History of Testosterone Research

So you don't want your sex life to come to an end. You want to stay focused and healthy. You've found that testosterone is the key. You're well on your way to discovering exactly what many scientists and medical professionals learned years ago.

Ancient cultures have a long history of documenting the differences between men and women but that difference was only demonstrated by indicating the differences between genitalia. Ancient cultures were not so far off when they pointed to the testicles as the source of maleness but they had no way of identifying testosterone – let alone preserving it.

It wasn't until 1935 that a Dutch researcher managed to put a name to testosterone and shortly thereafter that that the location of this substance became known. You see, as Croatian researcher Leopold Ruzicka pointed out, although the testicles possess some testosterone (certainly at convenient times), they are not testosterone's *raison d'être*.

Ruzicka made it clear to the world that testosterone is used throughout the body and the bloodstream must deliver it to all the parts of the body that receive it. Moreover, an effective supply of testosterone must be maintained.

Ruzicka is also credited with being the first man to produce synthetic testosterone, using cholesterol and trial and error until he found the formula. Once he succeeded, his research led to widespread commercial production of synthetic testosterone.

Despite the desire to continue along the same lines of Ruzicka's replication research, it was soon revealed as an impractical approach. Fellow researchers discovered that the use of effective amounts of this synthetic testosterone would significantly harm the liver.

This is because the liver acts as a filtration system for the body. Since everything orally ingested must pass through the liver, the liver filtered out much of the synthetically administered testosterone before it could have any of the desired effects.

Researchers hoped that by injecting synthetic testosterone, they could bypass liver function. However, the injections were painful and required too much frequency to be a practical solution to a lack of testosterone.

As research looked for the most practical line for testosterone bolstering, pharmaceutical companies looked for the most profitable method of testosterone building – and soon found what they sought in a pill. The industry began mass producing bulk amounts of synthetic testosterone to 'help its users" despite the practicality issues uncovered by researchers.

3. Cialis, Levitra, Staxyn, and Viagra: Big Pharma's Four Pillars of Testosterone

The four pills that can save a man - these trademarked products have earned big money for their makers. These drugs are FDA approved and tend to treat some of the problems that frequently afflict those with low testosterone. However, they may cause a variety of side effects.

What are the side effects?
Cialis – 36 hours ("the weekender")
Levitra and Staxyn – 5 hours
Viagra – 4 hours

Headaches, rashes or an itching sensation, heartburn, chest pain, stomach problems, back pain, blurred vision, heart attacks and drug interactions with other medications are all reactions cited by the users of these drugs. Should you take certain blood pressure medications or nitroglycerin and you ingest one of these drugs, it can cause even more serious prostate issues or serious crises of blood pressure.

Along with the physiological side effects of these pills, there is also the psychological side effect that unfortunately occurs when you take your "little blue pill" only to find your partner unwilling. You now have a $10 erection that means nothing with corresponding embarrassment and disappointment to boot.

Note: The exception to the 'disappointment issue' is of course Cialis because this drug is taken in anticipation of sex over a 36 hour period (the others need to be taken one hour before anticipated sex).

In fact, these drugs can't even be taken by some people.

Who can't take these drugs?

- People with high blood pressure or low blood pressure
- People with chest pains during intercourse
- People with angina
- People who have suffered a stroke, heart attack or cardiac arrhythmia within six months of taking the drug

Should you wonder if you're a candidate for this list, seek the opinion of a professional medical practitioner who can answer your concerns.

These drugs are touted as the solution to men's testosterone deficiency but in truth their effectiveness is often outweighed by the risk to the patient. They are only temporary solutions to a seemingly 'permanent' problem and should not be relied upon for the long term.

4. Temporary, Dangerous Solutions

When these drugs first appeared they were greeted with enthusiasm from the medical community. Researchers in 1942 discovered that those taking these drugs felt completely alleviated of their andropause symptoms (lack of energy, depression, memory blanks, trouble sleeping and poor self-esteem) within a few weeks. The research looked great, but beneficiary effects of the drugs were only temporary. We now understand why.

The body always seeks to maintain balance. When you inject a supply of one substance, synthetic or not, the body will lower its production of that substance to compensate. This is what happened with testosterone injections. The bodies of the men taking these drugs would initially spike in testosterone but then begin to compensate for the injections by producing less. This means the injections were only able to keep the same problematic level of testosterone for just a short time after they were "working."

You may be thinking this problem could be solved with increased dosages but this solution doesn't work either. When the body is first offered synthetic testosterone it reduces its own production but when dosages are increased it eventually shuts down receptors within the body for testosterone altogether. This is to say nothing of the side effects of synthetic testosterone injections, which are dangerous enough.

This unfortunate discovery was made by athletes who used steroids to improve their performance. By 1960 it was finally determined that, much like orally ingested testosterone, injections can result in serious liver damage and even long term liver disease. Want to exchange jaundice, cancer or hepatitis for andropause? Didn't think so.

In the aftermath of these damaging discoveries, anti-steroid campaigns spread like wildfire, raising an outcry for the prohibition of steroids. In 1990 the United States Congress amended the Controlled Substance Act designating anabolic steroids as a Schedule III drug, requiring a health practitioner's prescription for its use and possession.

Despite the clamor for stricter controls on steroids, research continues on testosterone (a steroid) and its effects, with many still touting its benefits.

5. The Positive Effects of Testosterone

"People have noticed a change. I can stride confidently, knowing I am ready for that business meeting and that I will succeed."

This is an example of how testosterone positively affected a 40 year old business executive. Increasing his testosterone levels increased his motivation and most importantly, his confidence. He is not the only one who has been positively impacted.

"I was having trouble sleeping and controlling my weight. I was depressed and I always seemed to be so tired. I now weigh 185lbs, I haven't taken a nap in ages and I have had the energy to start reaching some of my fitness goals of working out more often. Let me tell you, this feels GOOD. I feel alive!"

The above story is an effective testimonial to the effects of testosterone. The author actually was suffering not just from lack of testosterone, but also from the effects of HIV. By increasing his testosterone levels he was able to achieve positive changes in his life.

Below is a summary of significant research findings regarding testosterone:

- Dr. Randall Urban of the University of Texas at Galveston linked testosterone with the positive effects of increased sex drive, increased muscular size and strength without added workout exercises. He also found that testosterone infused men with vigor and youthful joy.

- Dr. Dana Ohl, co-director of the University of Michigan's Center for Fertility and Sexuality, performed a review highlighting the findings of several research studies. Testosterone therapy was linked to an increased ability to make reasonable decisions, increased muscular body mass, increased strength and decreased levels of unhealthy fat.

- Dr. Fred Sexton of the University of Western Ontario found that by helping the body to produce more testosterone you can help reverse symptoms of andropause including lack of sex drive, emotional instability, lack of self-esteem and loss of muscular strength and form.

- Dr. Darryl O'Conner of the United Kingdom published findings to the British Psychological Society showing testosterone levels are positively linked with language skills (the higher your testosterone is, the higher your language skills will be).

- The University of Cambridge published a study in 2008 which included testing 17 stock market day traders (via their saliva) two times a day for a little over a week. Their findings? Not surprisingly, those higher in testosterone made significantly higher returns than those who had lower levels, linking testosterone to a bigger paycheck!

- Healthy (higher) levels of testosterone are directly correlated with lower levels of LDL (bad cholesterol) and higher levels of HDL (healthy cholesterol).

- The National Osteoporosis Foundation has declared that lower testosterone levels are associated with bone loss and osteoporosis

Testosterone therapy has an effect, and it can be far reaching. A student in Dr. Randall Urban's study was so transformed by the results of this therapy that he literally had to stop taking testosterone interventions during exams due to the distracting presence of his now rampant sexual desires!

But what does all of this research mean for you?

6. There Is Hope

"*There is no other substance on the planet, natural or man-made, that can have such profound effects*" Dr. Karlis Ullis, M.D., author of 'Super T'

We have shown the positive effects of testosterone. It can increase muscle mass, strengthen your bones, help you sleep better and restore the ability to focus and elevate your confidence. The "he hormone" has made nearly miraculous changes in the lives of many men.

Unfortunately, we also know the side effects of testosterone injections and the fleeting benefits of testosterone's 'miracle pills.' These therapies can be costly and time consuming, two detriments to the ability to recover from andropause.

Thankfully, there is an alternative -- the natural method. What the body does naturally is often best, and there are definitely ways to naturally increase your testosterone production.

The other great news? This increase doesn't just help to prevent these problems. It can undo a lot of the damage that a lack of testosterone has done. Whether you're in your 20s and looking to take better care of yourself or in your 40s and in the throes of andropause, there is a solution – seek to boost your testosterone *naturally*.

The following chapters will demonstrate how to naturally boost your testosterone and the steps to take to affect its positive change in your life.

THERE IS HOPE!

Boosting Your Testosterone Levels – The Natural Way

Natural methods of boosting testosterone are often best because they incorporate your body in combating the effects of a testosterone deficiency and thus increase your chances of having long term success. If you want to take a natural approach there are steps you can take.

As any doctor worth their medical license will tell you, health issues are never just limited to an immediate problem. They also include factors that lead to the problem. Diet, physical activity, even your emotional state – are all critical factors in keeping you healthy (both mentally and physically).

The best advice is to attack the problem on all fronts. Not only will you make changes in your lifestyle, you will also incorporate the research of multiple disciplines to affect these changes. In other words, don't depend on one approach to make the difference in your life.

What's To Come – A Chapter Overview of the Strategy:

- **Section I: Self-Assessment**
  A self-assessing questionnaire that will reveal your current testosterone level.

- **Section II: What Can Impact Your Testosterone**
  What can get in the way of improving your testosterone levels and what to do about it.

- **Section III: Herbal Methods to Increase Your Testosterone**
  From supplements to vitamins, herbs can play a big role controlling your bodily production of hormones.

- **Section IV: How Your Diet Impacts Your Testosterone**
  This section details the importance of your diet with your testosterone level, and how to know what foods will help.

- **Section V: Sex, the Ultimate Testosterone Boost**
  You may not be aware of this, but it's an extremely helpful (and fun) way to boost your testosterone.

- **Section VI: Weight Loss, the Testosterone Solution?**
  Ways to lose weight while you're working at self-improvement including a sample of a food diary, tips and a fat storing, high glycemic index.

- **Section VII: The Importance of Physical Activity**
  How will you know what you're doing is working? This section will overview the signs of success.

- **Section VIII: When Will You See Results?**
  Types of exercise to support your body physically, in terms of strength, flexibility and heart health.

- **Conclusions**
  After all this you'll be prepared to get started. This section will summarize some of the things we've learned and provide you with a questionnaire again to assess your levels of testosterone.

Section I: Self-Assessment

This assessment is a tool to help you evaluate if you are currently at an acceptable level of testosterone. Don't be afraid to be honest; you can get results no matter what you score.

	Frequently	Occasionally	Never
	1	2	3
1. Do you have trouble obtaining an erection?			
2. Do you lose your erection before orgasm?			
3. When attempting sexual intercourse how often is it unsatisfactory for you?			
4. Have you noticed a decreased interest in sex?			
5. Do you drink alcohol?			
6. Do you smoke tobacco?			
7. Do you find yourself with a lack of ambition and motivation?			
8. Do you lack the energy to climb a short flight of stairs?			
9. Do you find yourself becoming moody, depressed or irritable without good reason?			

10. How often do you find yourself lacking the strength to lift a heavy household object like a full garbage can?			
11. How often do you lack the desire to get up in the morning?			
12. How often are you disinterested in exercising?			
13. How many prescription drugs do you regularly take?	3 or More	1 – 2	None
14. Pinch your fat just to the side of your belly button. How much can you pinch?	> 1”	About 1”	< 1”
15. What is your age?	> 50	35 – 50	< 35
TOTAL:			
	x 0	x 5	x 10

SCORING:

- Score 0 points for each response in column 1
- 5 points for each response in column 2
- 10 points for each response in column 3

POINTS: ______

ANALYSIS:

Over 125 = FABULOUS

You're doing great! Keep up the good work.

100 – 125 = AVERAGE

You're doing okay but you could benefit from testosterone boosting techniques to both protect what you still have and possibly recover some that may be lost.

Below 100 = DEFICIENT

You may among those who are already suffering from extremely depleted testosterone levels and would definitely benefit from testosterone boosting.

If you scored worse than you thought...

Don't be surprised. Testosterone is not something we think to check, even when we suffer from many symptoms of a deficiency. One reason this has reached an epidemic level is men don't check these things out. Remember, there are a lot of other men just like you who suffer without fully understanding why.

Testosterone deficiencies can be addressed and your symptoms can improve!

Section II: What Can Impact Your Testosterone?

There are many factors you may not think would impact your body that actually affect your testosterone levels. These rascals work hard to decrease your hormone levels even as you work hard to elevate them. So what factors are the most important? Consider the following list.

- Alcohol - is a drug but not one we typically group with prescriptions or antibiotics, so it will be handled separately. The main point with alcohol -- moderate your drinking. No matter what a 22 year old may think, alcohol is a leading cause of a host of medical issues, including impotence. Nothing slows an erection more than "just a few beers."

- Junk food – a topic most of us would prefer to avoid. Who doesn't love their coffee in the morning? The truth is that caffeine and sugar are two of the most nefarious testosterone thieves. If you can take coffee with a little less sugar, it will help. If you can have one coke a week instead of one every hour, that will help. Can you substitute your unhealthy drinking habits with water? That will help *tremendously.*

- Drugs – whether legal or illegal, prescription or over the counter -- greatly impact your body. While some effects can be obvious (making you feel better, inducing recovery, etc.) you need to be aware that they also impact your testosterone levels. This doesn't mean you can never take another antibiotic; it just means you shouldn't ingest Tylenol every five minutes.

  A particularly nasty list of drugs is included below to show just how vast their impact can be.

- Romantic dinners – This is an odd one to be sure, but it seems to be related to gluttony. When you're stuffing your face with a full three course meal, and you only needed one of those courses, it slows your body down – and rapidly decreases testosterone. Even if you can maintain an erection after a big meal, it's not normally as hard (or big!) as when your body is working at peak efficiency. Overindulging when it comes to food also leads to a host of medical problems such as heart disease, obesity and arteriosclerosis.

1. Prescriptions and Food Additives Make a Huge Difference in Your Sex Life

The following drugs in particular have been implicated in the reduction of sex drive and thus should only be taken as needed.

Adrenergic blockers; two types

- Alpha-blockers: phentolamine (Regitine) phenoxybenzaimine (Dibenzyline) prazosin (Minizide)
- Beta-blockers: Digoxin (Lanoxin, Lanoxicaps), propanolol (Inderal), metoprolol (Toprol) atenolol (Tenormin)
- Calcium Channel Blockers: amlodipine (Norvasc), amlodipine/ atorvastatin (Caduet), amlodine/benazepril (Lotrel), amlodipine/ valsartan (Exforge), Cardizem, diltiazem,felodipine (Plendil), isradipine, nicardipine (Cardene), nifedipine (Adalat, Procardia), disopyramide (Norpace) verapamil (Calan, Verelan, Isoptin SR)
- Central Sympatholytics *(treatment of high blood pressure through central nervous system):* clonidine (Catapres) guanabenz (Wytensin) guanfacine (Tenex) reserpine (Diupres) methyldopa (Aldoclor)
- Mixed blockers: labetalol (Trandate)

Antacids:

- *Cimetidine (Tagamet)*
- *Famotidine (Pepcid)*
- *Ranitidine*

Anti-Asthmatics Primarily ephedrine (Quadrinal)

Anticholinergics

- Atropine (Donnatal)
- Benztropine (Cogentin)
- Diphenhydramine (Benadryl)
- Propantheline (Pro-Banthine)

Antidepressants

- MAO inhibitors — phenelzine (Nardil), isocarboxiazid (Marplan) tranyleypromine (Pamate) procarbazine (Matulane)
- Tricyclics — amitriptyline (Elavil) desipramine (Norproamin) nortriptyline (Pamelor) doxepin (Adapin) clomiproamine (Anafranil)

Anti-DHT Hair Loss / Prostate Hypertrophy Drug

- finasteride (Propecia, Proscar)

Anti-Fungal

- ketoconazole (Nizoral)

Antihypertensives (often used to treat high blood pressure)

- Adrenergic antagonists *(treat high blood pressure and benign prostate disease)*: guanethidine (Esimil) guanadrel (Hylorel) mecamylamine (Inversine)
- Loop diuretics: furosemide (Lasix), bumetanide (Bumex), ethacrynic acid (Edecrin)
- Potassium-sparing diuretics: spironolactone (Aldactone), amiloride (Midamor), triamterene (Dyazide)
- Thiazide diuretics: hydrochlorothiazide, Aldactazide, chlorthalidone (Combipres)

Anxiolytics

- Anti-anxiety drugs: diazepam (Valium) chlorazepate, chlordiazepoxide (Librium), triazolam (Halcion)

Benzodiazepines (tranquilizers)

*List includes only the most commonly prescribed

- Alprazolam (Xanax, Xanor, Kalma, Tafil, Alprox, Frontal(Brazil),
- Chlordiazepoxide (Librium, Tropium, Risolid, Klopoxid)
- Clonazepam (Klonopin, Klonapin, Rivotril)
- Clorazepate (Tranxene)
- Diazepam (Valium)
- Estazolam (ProSom)
- Flunitrazepam (Rohypnol, Rohydorm (Brazil)
- Flurazepam (Dalmane)
- Lorazepam (Ativan, Temesta, Lorabenz)
- Medazepam (Nobrium)
- Midazolam (Dormicum, Versed, Hypnovel, Dormonid (Brazil)
- Oxazepam (Seresta, Serax, Serenid, Serepax, Sobril, Oxascand, Alopam, Oxabenz, Oxapax, Murelax, Alepam
- Phenazepam (Russia)
- Quazepam (Doral)
- Temazepam (Restoril, Normison, Euhypnos Nocturne, Temaze or Temtabs)
- Triazolam (Halcion, Rilamir)

Carbonic anhydrase inhibitors

- Acetazolamide (Diamox)
- Methazolamide

Environmental

- Bisphenol A (BPA): leaches into food/drink from storing in plastics.
- Lead: paint, structures in houses built before 1960 could contain lead.

- Mercury: replace tooth fillings with new composites.
- Pesticides: fruits, vegetables, plants. Wash carefully. Buy organic.
- Phthalates: chemicals used in household spray deodorants, plastic toys.

Excitotoxins

- Monosodium glutamate, autolyzed yeast food additives (glutamate, hydrolyzed protein, sodium caseinate). Aspartame (artificial sweetener marketed as Equal). *Some Rx drugs contain excitotoxins; ask your pharmacist.

Recreational Drugs

- Alcohol, Amphetamines, barbiturates, benzodiazepines, cocaine, Ecstasy, heroin, LSD, marijuana, mescaline, methamphetamine, opium, psychedelic mushrooms, solvent sniffing, tobacco.

Sedatives

- Barbiturates
- Meprobamate (Deprol)

Statins (drugs prescribed to lower cholesterol)

- Crestor, Lipitor, atorvastatin, simvastatin, rosuvastatin

Tranquilizers

- Butyrophenones: haloperidol (Haldol) Phenothiazines chlorpromazine (Thorazine) mesoridazine (Serentil) Thioxanthenos chlorprothixene (Taractan) thiothixene (Navane)

Vasodilators

- Hydralazine (Ser-Ap-Es)

These drugs may include some lifestyle factors you've already considered. On the other hand, they may be a complete shock to you. Nonetheless, they all have one commonality – they threaten your testosterone levels. These are not the only factors, as there is one large factor we have not yet addressed.

2. Stress

Stress is something we all deal with at some point. Ask your doctor, ask your mother, ask your wife, they'll all say the same thing – and even you know this is true. It's an all too familiar feeling; the frustration is just too much and you feel as if your head will explode.

The problem is that stress has an effect on the body even beyond your mental anxiety. Stress has been shown to raise blood pressure, wreck your hormones (including testosterone), lead to weight gain and weaken your immune system. These effects cannot be ignored. For the sake of your health and for the sake of your testosterone levels, the repercussions cannot be ignored either.

By recognizing stress we can work to counteract its effects. How do we do that?

- Accept that stress will happen. This recognition will enable you to move forward as you compartmentalize the effects of stress and will prepare you for its impact before it arises.

- Learn to recognize the signs that you're stressed. If you know what to look for, you can learn how to prepare yourself before stress hits. Stress will happen -- you need to be not only prepared for it mentally, but also know how to handle it physically.

- Know what helps calm you when you're stressed!

Ways to Reduce Stress

Tibetan monks are famous for their ability to completely avoid stress (and pain and other distractions). People have great admiration for their ability to deal with stress. While their dedication to their cause is admirable, monks are not the only ones with this ability.

There are a lot of ways to reduce stress -- beginning a new hobby, reading a book, listening to music or taking a hot bath. The point is that since no two people are exactly alike, you should find what stress reduction method specifically works *for you.* And then practice it regularly.

The following are a series of simple techniques that often reduce stress for people and are great places to start if you have no idea what can calm you.

3. Take a Cleansing Breath

This is one your mom probably taught you, and one that has remarkably visible effects. Take a deep breath through your nose and hold it for a few seconds before slowly allowing yourself to exhale. This exhalation purges your body of stress; feel it leave your body with the rush of air billowing from your lungs and how you've changed your outlook.

This is a simple, but extremely effective exercise that obviously can be done as often (or as seldom) as needed!

4. Take a Moment Off and Give Yourself a Break

Say your boss has just started yelling again. Or you spilled coffee all over your new pants. Or you just can't sleep. What do you do?

Take a few minutes to let yourself genuinely relax. This means allowing yourself to sit in a comfortable position or lay down. Focusing on breathing deeply in and out; you should feel it in your abdomen. Sense how that breath impacts your body. Don't be distracted by what's going on around you but rather focus exclusively on how the air moves throughout your body.

You should do this exercise daily for 10 to 20 minutes at a time when possible. From a practical standpoint, do it whenever needed!

5. Fixing Your Posture

This is another exceedingly simple and seemingly small way to dramatically reduce your stress level.

How do you do it? While sitting in a chair, take a moment to consider your posture.

1) Your shoulders should be extremely relaxed. You can recognize this state of relaxation when you feel no strain throughout the neck or shoulders. When you have relaxed your shoulders, drop your arms to the sides of your body (they deserve a break too).

2) Lay your hands palms up on your lap.

3) Gently shift your legs so that your knees are bent only to the point of comfort and your feet are in front of you, comfortably extended.

4) Take a deep breath, allowing even your mouth to relax.

This exercise can be repeated as desired and is definitely a great stress buster!

6. Meditation

What it is? Another technique, inducing a calming state to the point that it impacts your attitude.

How do you do it?

1) Set the stage for an effective meditation. This means finding a quiet room where you can sit in silence and be alone without distraction.

2) Relax your body. Breathe in slowly and breathe out. Stretch if it helps to relax your muscles. The calmer your body is, the easier it will be for you to focus and meditate efficiently.

3) Meditation is centered on the idea of meditating on some concept or object. Hence, the first step is to find something you'd like to focus on -- maybe peace, maybe happiness or maybe just relaxation. Whatever it is, you need to focus on it for a while for meditation to work.

4) Focus on the mantra you have chosen. Clear your mind except for the mantra, remaining as passive as possible about whether it's "working or not."

How long should you do this exercise to receive its benefits? Meditate for 10 - 20 minutes at a time, and it can easily be incorporated into your daily routine for maximum effect.

7. Let the Little Things Go!

Stress happens to all of us and it happens quite frequently. Realize that a lot of what we stress over is actually a lot less important than how it feels at the time. Take a minute and consider the big picture. Is this really going to impact your life? What's the worst outcome of this occurrence?

By putting matters into perspective you will calm yourself even before trying another stress reduction technique.

8. Remove Yourself If Necessary

If you really feel your blood starting to boil, it's not going to help your body to scream. If none of the above techniques are working at this moment, remove yourself from the situation. This could mean taking a walk, taking a bath, walking into another room -- you just need to take a few minutes to calm yourself again.

The Take Home Message

The real take home message is to find what works for you and use it to calm yourself as often as possible. Stress negatively impacts the body in a dramatic way. This includes your testosterone levels as well as your heart's health.

Put things into perspective, take a deep breath and don't be afraid to take a moment or two off if you need a break – we all do sometimes. When you pay attention to your body and handle stress efficiently, you will notice a dramatic quality of life improvement. It's an added bonus as you increase your testosterone levels!

9. Other Issues That Can Impact Your Testosterone

Although there are several factors that you can control (i.e., alcohol intake, drug usage, etc.), some of your bodily organs -- which you cannot necessarily control -- can impact your testosterone levels. The following is a list detailing some of the conditions that can affect your levels of testosterone and how to recognize which ones afflict you.

Trans Fats

Trans fats are food preservatives that confound your testosterone levels. Why? Trans fats are high in LDL (bad cholesterol) and low in HDL (good cholesterol). We've already briefly discussed this effect but bad cholesterol clogs your arteries, which causes difficulties in maintaining erections and with your body's ability to balance itself.

Overly Rigid Dieting

A healthy diet is important, and dieting has its place, but too often people indulge in overly rigid diets that promise quick results – and end up not only failing, but depleting their testosterone levels. This is because when you slow your metabolism down you also weaken your hypothalamus, the part of the brain that directs the pituitary (center for hormone production). It's also impacted by the fact that diets tend to focus on reducing various animal fats yet these substances actually increase your testosterone production.

You can diet in a healthy way and still avoid harming your testosterone. You just have to be careful. We will discuss this more in detail later.

The Liver

The liver is an organ that acts as a filter, as we said earlier. It removes excessive substances within the body. This is great when it works, but when it doesn't it only serves to aggravate hormonal imbalance. The liver's health is often a result of what we put into our bodies. Treatment for a liver problem is usually a liver detox followed by a healthier lifestyle regimen.

One liver detox program calls for drinking a glass of hot water with lemon juice and a tablespoon of olive oil every day for a week.

Other substances that help cleanse the liver include water, milk thistle, marshmallow root and other herbs.

To protect your liver avoid excessive use of alcohol, herbs that damage the liver and excessive use of acetaminophen.

The Thyroid

The thyroid is the organ responsible for the production of androgens and estrogens for the body. This is an important organ because if it is off kilter your testosterone levels will be too.

Symptoms of a thyroid problem:

- Fatigue
- Depression
- Rapid weight gain
- Erection maintenance issues

If your doctor identifies you as having a thyroid problem he will most likely treat it by supplementing your hormone levels and informing you of dietary steps you can take to improve the function of your thyroid.

The reason that diet comes into play is because the thyroid is affected by what you eat. Typical foods to avoid will be discussed later in the book but include soy. Thyroid-enhancing foods include those high in selenium and iodine.

A Good Night's Sleep is absolutely necessary to improve your levels of testosterone. Why? Sleep is a time for regeneration. Your body actually creates needed hormones that and begins working to rejuvenate itself. When you aren't sleeping well, or often enough, studies have shown your testosterone levels could be as low as 20% of what it should be! So make sure you get quality sleep.

10. Conclusion

Each of these factors impacts your testosterone in some way and each of them can be managed. If you take into account the tips provided here you will be well on your way to a naturally healthier level of testosterone – and a happier life.

Summary of Advice to Make the Lowest Possible Testosterone Impact

- Avoid using drugs when you can – this includes everything from prescriptions to recreational, as drugs in general have a negative impact. Please note that there are some cases where you will need drugs for illness. In this case they should not be avoided.

  Use your judgment and find a doctor you trust. Make him/her aware that you're trying to avoid these drugs unless necessary. They often will work with you in conjunction with your health goals, and if they won't, see if there is a reason. If they are unwilling to accommodate your wishes, consider consulting another physician regarding the use of the drugs in question.

- Don't let stress get the better of you. Learn what stresses you and how to avoid it or manage it. Discover your favorite stress-relieving technique and use it as often as needed!

- Get examined if you've addressed the issues above and still suffer from low testosterone. A medical professional will be able to better assess your condition, such as issues with your liver or thyroid. Knowledge is a huge help in the battle to raise testosterone levels.

- Avoid excessively rigid diets that can often hurt you more than help.

- Every night make sure to get a good night's sleep! Never underestimate your body's powers of rejuvenation by depriving yourself of the opportunity for satisfying and complete rest.

Section III: Herbal Methods to Increase Your Testosterone

Even with all the steps you've taken, you sometimes need supplements to recover your testosterone. It's important to work as naturally as you can to stimulate your body's production. With that in mind, consider the following tips for natural production:

- If you are currently struggling with obesity, look into supplements that can help you to lose weight healthily. Consider chromium polynicotinate, an ionic substance that requires a starting dosage of 200 micrograms a day, gradually moving to 800 mg. In six weeks you should be seeing noticeable results.

- Begin to make use of multivitamins and mineral supplements as necessary.

- If you are 40 years of age or older, add antioxidant supplements like Vitamins C, D and E, selenium and CoQ10 to your dietary regimen.

These are some of the supplements that can start you on your path but there are several more that will naturally aid your body in producing the "He Hormone." This chapter will walk you through some of the most effective herbal solutions and why they work so well.

However, before we begin, let's consider the impact of estrogen.

1. The Issues of Estrogen

Many people assume that testosterone is a bad hormone, responsible for aggression and violence, but this is not the case. Testosterone is also associated with cognitive abilities (your ability to reason and focus), stay fit (helps the body to build muscles) and keeps a normal and healthy level of sexual desire flowing through your system. We've talked at length about the numerous benefits of testosterone, which affects your body on many more levels than just aggression.

Your testosterone levels are declining. The level of testosterone in your body peaks in your 20s and as you age, testosterone levels continue to decline. Yet testosterone deficiency is not your only cause for concern.

We've learned a lot about a lack of testosterone and what can impact your testosterone levels but andropause is not the only issue you face. The threat to your manhood is more than just a lack of testosterone; the estrogen within your body can dominate your system with greater ease as you age.

The male body normally contains a minimal level of estrogen and (hopefully) a healthy level of testosterone. Normally, testosterone dominates estrogen in the male body, which manifests itself through virilization. But if estrogen can gain the upper hand, where does it come from?

It is a common misconception that estrogen is "just" a female hormone. Though estrogen is associated with typically feminine characteristics, and testosterone with masculinity, there are levels of both in each gender. Estrogen is present in food, the air and even in the liquids you consume. Your body can amass a storehouse of the hormone while you remain unaware of the accumulation.

The key is balance between estrogen and testosterone. In a typical female, estrogen will outweigh testosterone several times over and vice versa for males. However, aging reduces the hormone ratio in men.

As you age you lose testosterone. We've discussed this at length but now consider the fact that your estrogen levels are rising. Part of your andropause problem is that as you lose testosterone the ratio between the two hormones becomes skewed. Thus the effects of estrogen begin to dominate your body while those of testosterone stop working.

You may wonder about the significance of a higher estrogen levels in your body. Let's look at some of its effects and you can decide for yourself:

- Moodiness
- Lower muscular mass
- Muscular atrophy (a decrease in muscular mass)
- Weight gain
- Lowered sex drive

Still not convinced? The male body is not intended to be dominated by estrogen. Fortunately, this chapter will review the available literature on how you can keep estrogen levels to a minimum so you can combat this imbalance.

As we examine the research we will identify beneficial supplements and their effective use. We also provide advice on how to recognize your proper dosage. Best of all, we will help you control this condition before it even starts.

2. Ways to Minimize Estrogen

The most efficient way to control the level of estrogen in your body is through supplements. Supplements work with your body to maintain balance between testosterone and estrogen at healthy, normal levels. It should be noted that when we talk about supplements we do not necessarily mean pills. Supplementary substances can be ingested through the food you eat just as easily as a popping a pill in the morning. In fact it is better for you to add supplements from your diet rather than pills.

That said, there are two primary supplements that must be discussed in terms of estrogen control: Indole-3-Carbinol and DIM.

Indole-3-Carbinol

Recommended daily dosage: 200 mg.

Indole-3-Carbinol is a supplement that can either be taken in pill form or by ingestion of cruciferous vegetables. For those of us needing a vocabulary refresher, cruciferous vegetables tend to be 'green' ones (asparagus, kale, broccoli, Brussels sprouts, cauliflower and others).

Indole-3-Carbinol has been linked not only to the control of estrogen but to protection from cancer. Estrogen contributes to tumor growth so by dissipating this hormone you decrease your risks.

DiIndolylMethane (DIM)

Recommended daily dosage: 200-400mg daily (in supplements or from cruciferous vegetables).

Several years ago, DIM supplements were evaluated in a UC Berkeley study that tested the urine levels of participants. Their findings? Estrogen levels were significantly lower in the urine of those who took DIM supplements than in those who did not.

Estrogen control is also not the only benefit DIM provides. The Department of Molecular and Cell Biology at UC Berkeley also found in a separate study that DIM slows the growth of cancer cells by as much as 70%! A diet rich in foods with DIM has been shown to be an effective regimen for cancer patients as well.

DIM is a supplement that naturally works with the body to metabolize estrogen (breaking it down into more useful blocks for your body). It is present in a number of foods, primarily "green" vegetables (cauliflower, asparagus, broccoli, and cabbage – even Brussels sprouts!)

Please note that if you are supplementing your diet with cruciferous vegetables and you have a thyroid condition, you must steam the vegetables first. Raw vegetables contain compounds that can make it difficult for your body to access the effects of your thyroid medications.

Estrogen control is not the only part to this puzzle

While ensuring that your estrogen levels are minimized is a critical part of battling andropause, it is critical that when supplement your diet you do not forget to raise your levels of testosterone. Having higher levels of testosterone and lower levels of estrogen is your body's best shot at remaining the man you want to be for as long as possible.

3. Ways to Boost Testosterone

Before 1997, men who looked for help with the "normal signs of aging" (difficulty maintaining erections, loss of muscle mass, reduction of sex drive) had only diet and exercise to rely on. Doctors knew that testosterone injections would cause more harm than good and had limited options available to countermand the effects of aging. This has changed.

We have some great news. Although medical history has consistently showed the impracticality of taking testosterone injections to maintain your testosterone levels, research has recently discovered a potentially natural solution -- testosterone precursors.

Now the substances that promote the production of testosterone have been identified. Specifically, the chemicals that increase testosterone within your own body (naturally) have been found. This means you can boost your testosterone naturally without needing direct injections or even ingesting supplements!

This is a huge breakthrough because we now have access to information regarding affordable testosterone-inducing substances available to you – without needing a doctor's prescription. Even better, these substances work naturally within the body – increasing your chance of long term success in raising your testosterone!

So what should you be taking?

At first researchers were finding the most success with androstenedione supplements, made famous by MLB home run king Mark McGuire. These supplements, as suggested by the name, produce the andros hormones that help you to feel virile. They can raise your testosterone levels by as much as 183%. You may note the disclaimer "at first," and here's why. As of April 2004, the FDA banned OTC usage of "Andro," requiring a prescription for its use. Thus it is not readily available to the men who need it most. However, researchers have found other options that are still available today.

DeHyroEpiAndrosterone (DHEA)

Recommended daily dosage: The typical course of treatment is 10 mg daily, increasing as necessary. Your daily dosage of DHEA will depend on a number of factors related to your current levels of certain hormones and what your personal optimal levels are. Seek medical attention before taking a DHEA supplement.

NOTE: DHEA should only be taken by men who are low in this hormone. This is why medical attention is so critical. Much like cortisol (discussed below), a little is great but too much is bad for you. Work with your medical professional to keep your DHEA levels at a healthy level for you – this will have the optimal effect.

DHEA may be a 'runner up' in efficacy to androstenedione but it is legal and safe (unlike its FDA banned counterpart). It is an extremely effective tool to boost your testosterone because it is a naturally occurring substance within the body.

What this means is that your body already contains DHEA within. In fact, it's one of the top hormones that your body produces. Like testosterone however, your DHEA levels decrease with age. By the time you qualify for senior discounts, you've already lost 90% of your body's ability to produce DHEA and thus the testosterone to which it can be converted.

DHEA can be converted to a number of bodily substances; it's what your body turns to when low on hormones. As such, it provides many health benefits to your body in addition to supplementing your testosterone levels. What are some of these benefits? Weight loss, an increase in insulin balance, healthier connective tissues, a sense of overall happiness and life satisfaction and a reduction of stress – arguably leading to an even longer list of health benefits.

In addition to lowering stress levels, DHEA reduces cortisol, a stress hormone that can wreak havoc on your body if left unchecked. It should be noted that in small doses cortisol is beneficial – it stimulates your fight-or-flight response and the survival instinct so familiar to us all. The problem is when you're not in danger and cortisol is present, it interferes with the body's daily drive to not just survive but to thrive. This is what you observe in people who are chronically stressed -- the worrywart type who always frets.

Other benefits of DHEA include increased memory capacity, fewer instances of illness, higher performance on both physical and mental tests and less fat content within the body. It also promotes retention of that youthful glow we all wish we still had.

The following lists some of the research findings connected with the medical benefits of DHEA:

- Researchers at the University of Vienna found that healthy DHEA levels were strongly linked to the ability to maintain an erection and increased sex drive.

- Russian researchers found that patients low in DHEA often suffered from sexual issues such as erectile dysfunction and a reduced sex drive. Conversely, patients high in DHEA had great success at erection formation and maintenance and maintained a healthy sex drive.

- The Institute of Biomedical Research at the University Of Birmingham, England found that DHEA improved sexual steroid levels in patients with impaired adrenal (hormone secretion) glands. This increase was associated with physical increases in energy, sex drive and mood.
- The University of Cambridge provided a meta-analytic review of the studies available on DHEA and well-being and found that 67% of patients in the studies who took DHEA did indeed report a significant improvement in life satisfaction.

A lot of problems attributed to aging are actually issues with lowered levels of testosterone and DHEA. DHEA is a great natural way to solve both of these hormonal problems and thus works to fight the issues that "aging" has supposedly brought. DHEA is not the only way to solve these problems. There are plenty of other natural testosterone-increasing substances that we now discuss.

4. Going Herbal – Herbal Remedies for Low Testosterone and Libidinal Issues

Herbs have been used long before man knew how to write down his ideas on how herbs could be used. All around the world we see evidence of people looking for that "magic plant" that will help them with their current ailments (ranging from illness to struggles with sexual dysfunction). Sexual dysfunction has resulted in a particularly passionate search.

There have been several herbs identified in the quest for prolonged sexual desire and performance throughout the aging process. Western medicine has unfortunately made a tradition out of rejecting the wisdom passed down from herb gatherers until very recently. Just because you are only now hearing about these herbs do not think they have been recently "discovered."

Herbs have a long history of both efficacy and safety. Simply put, if they caused harm to those who took them their usage would have ceased long ago. Just because Western medicine acknowledged their benefits only recently does not mean the use of herbs is new. It just points to the fact that Western medicine now recognizes their effectiveness.

In 1998 Americans witnessed a spending spike on natural herbs, supplements and vitamins. This surge was more profitable than the combined business done by pharmaceutical companies. The medical community decided to learn more about these substances if people were going to use them. Thus the hunt for the holistic remedy began.

Over time science and medicine have worked to identify the safest, most effective natural remedies. It is these remedies alone we will review.

Ashwagandha

Recommended daily dosage: 1 mg.

What is it?

Ayurvedic herbalists use Ashwagandha to treat sleeping disorders and chronic stress as well as libidinal issues.

How does it work?

It works to naturally teach the body to handle stress.

Avena Sativa

Recommended daily dosage: 50 mg.

What is it?

Avena Sativa, known as the common oat, is an alternative to erectile dysfunction treatment drugs.

How does it work?

Aveena Sativa breaks down testosterone into more mobile units, enabling it to reach more areas of the body. It also contains a psychoactive component that helps to calm the mind through its effects on the central nervous system. Whole oats can also lower cholesterol.

Citrulline

Recommended daily dosage: 1000 mg for up to 3 months at a time.

What is it?

Citrulline is an amino acid used to treat erectile dysfunction. A clinical study published from East Carolina University showed that those who took L-Citrulline at least twice a day experienced a significant increase in their levels of arginine of up to 65%, in just four weeks! Arginine, discussed later in this guide, helps then to directly produce testosterone.

How does it work?

Citrulline works with the body to break down arginine, allowing it to move swiftly throughout the small intestines.

Damiana

Recommended daily dosage: 100 mg.

NOTE: Diabetics should not be take damiana without consultation with a medical professional. This is because damiana has been known to interact with some diabetic medications and occasionally to lower blood sugar levels.

What is it?

Damiana, or *turnera diffusa*, is a herb found from southwestern Texas to South America and the Caribbean. It has been used for centuries to treat a host of medical issues including depression, diabetes, impotence, chronic stress, illnesses (bronchitis) and sexual dysfunction.

These effects have been validated by research, including an Italian study in 1999 which confirmed its success in treating sexual dysfunction. A 2002 U.S. patent was granted, based on the validity of medical findings concerning its restorative qualities, to a company that uses a proprietary blend of herbs including damiana.

When did we find it?

Damiana was recorded in the National Formulary in the United States in 1888 and included in several 19th century patent medicines. However, the ancient Maya and other Latin American cultures used the leaves as incense and as a tea with reputed aphrodisiac qualities. More recently, it is used as a component of a Mexican liqueur which in turn is an ingredient in traditional Mexican margaritas. Note that the state of Louisiana has outlawed its use and possession for human consumption.

Dopamine (L-Dopa)

Recommended daily dosage: 300 mg of an extract supplement containing at least 10% L-Dopa.

NOTE: You should not exceed the daily recommended dosage because if you do, you can experience feelings of hypersexuality. Hypersexuality will not kill you but can make you quite miserable. Just trust the recommended dosages and you will quickly see results – without seeing dangerous extreme ones.

What is it?

Dopamine is a neurotransmitter responsible for your brain's response to rewards and other pleasant sensations. It helps your body feel rewarded, thus encouraging you to repeat certain experiences, and is directly correlated to numerous aspects of your life – including your libido.

L-Dopa is synthetic dopamine; we suggest its use to supplement your libido and testosterone levels. L-Dopa was first created to treat Parkinson's disease. Subsequent research revealed its effects on sexually dysfunctional people.

You may wonder why we include a synthetic product in our "natural" section. This is because natural L-Dopa exists as well, largely in food items (like *mucuna pruriens* plant beans) and in supplements.

Epimedium

Recommended daily dosage: 250 - 500 mg

What is it?

Epimedium, Icariin or Horny Goat Weed, comes to us from the wisdom of ancient Chinese medicine. It is local to Asia and the Mediterranean.

Epimedium naturally enhances libido, which manifests itself both in erectile health and in stamina effects on your sex drive. *Epimedium* has also been used to treat joint problems as well as kidney and liver damage.

How does it work?

Like many of the herbs here, it makes testosterone increasingly mobile by breaking it down into smaller, more bodily accessible pieces. It also works to increase nitrous oxide levels, resulting in muscle relaxation and an increased flow of blood to the penis.

Interestingly, research is considering the possibility that *Epimedium* is also able to lower cortisol levels (which, if we recall from our earlier discussion, means higher DHEA and higher testosterone levels). Research is ongoing to translate Chinese wisdom into Western understanding of the herb but there is general consensus of its effects.

Eurycoma Longifolia

Recommended daily dosage: Half a capsule every day, increasing dosage slowly up to 1 capsule per day or every few days, as needed.

NOTE: Eurycoma Longifolia is associated with limited side effects of insomnia and irritability as well as an overall warmer body temperature. Thus it should only be taken with extreme caution in hot weather.

What is it?

Eurycoma Longifolia, or locally LongJax and Tongkat Ali, is native to the regions of Asia and Malaysia. It acts as an aphrodisiac and a natural strengthener for the body. Studies around the globe have found that Tonkkat Ali increases in libido and sexual behavior in as little as ten days.

Interestingly, in the study documenting the strengthening effects of LongJax, men who took the herb and participated in the same workout as men who did not take Longjax had increased significantly higher boosts to their performance in a strength contest. Moreover, those who took Longjax reduced their bodily fat content overall compared to those who did not.

How does it work?

Eurycoma Longifolia works to break down testosterone before it can be bound to receptors, enabling the smaller, more mobile pieces to reach more of the body before deactivating.

Ginkgo Biloba

Recommended daily dosage: 80 mg

What is it?

In 1989, Karlis Ullis, M.D. published a study within his book 'Super T' that displayed the power of Ginkgo to treat impotence. Over half of men tested completely restored their ability to create and maintain erections within six months of beginning use. This is only part of the effectiveness of Ginkgo.

This Chinese herb has been used for thousands of years not just to treat impotence but to treat the circulatory system (which also helps with erections and improves your health overall). Ginkgo is also an antioxidant, a substance known to assist with the restoration of memory and preservation of cognitive abilities (like focusing, multitasking, etc.).

How does it work?

Ginkgo works to boost the circulatory system, which allows healthier blood flow (and thus contributes to your ability to maintain erections. It even increases their quality).

Korean Ginseng

Recommended daily dosage: 100 - 200 mg of supplements containing at least 5 - 7% ginsenosides, taken in 3 week cycles (3 weeks on, 1 week off).

What is it?

Korean Ginseng is another Chinese herb that affects testosterone levels. It has been used as a health enhancer and has been found to increase the immune system, stamina and libido.

Muira Puama

Recommended daily dosage: 500 mg, two times daily.

NOTE: Has been known to increase insomnia if taken in excess

What is it?

Muira Puama, literally "potency wood," is a Brazilian herb traditionally used to treat a host of disorders including arthritis, rheumatism, impotence and dysentery.

Parisian wisdom has known about this herb since 1990 and the Institute of Sexology has documented the wonderful efficacy of Muira Puama as an aphrodisiac. Western medicine has shown that Muira Puama can be an extremely effective treatment for sufferers of erectile dysfunction. A 1990 study found a significance of 62% in treatment efficacy.

Saw Palmetto

Recommended daily dosage: 250 mg.

What is it?

Saw Palmetto is a Native American berry used to treat prostate disease, urinary issues and impotence.

As you age your testosterone decreases (as you know). This also causes an increase in DHT without production of testosterone, which can lead to excessive attachment to the prostate – and hyperplasia of prostate cells. Saw Palmetto slows the conversion rate of unused testosterone to DHT and works to prevent DHT from clogging up the prostate.

Tribulus Terrestris

Recommended daily dosage: 750 mg

What is it?

Tribulus Terrestris is one of the lesser known herbs for increasing testosterone levels. In Europe it is used to treat headaches and nervous disorders. These uses aside, Turkish, Ayurvedic and Oriental herbalists alike have all used *Tribulus Terrestris* to treat liver and kidney damage, cardiovascular diseases, blood pressure and impotence.

- The Bulgarian Medical Academy has confirmed its ability to aid the libido and act as an aphrodisiac.

- Indian researchers studied 50 people complaining of extensive exhaustion and trouble sleeping and found that almost half of those taking *Tribulus Terrestris* improved significantly within just a few days of beginning treatment.

    - Besides the benefits to sleep, 30% of those taking *Tribulus Terrestris* showed increased levels of blood which contributes to a number of positive health benefits.

- Singapore researchers who performed an eight week study on rats found that rats given *Tribulus Terrestris* showed signs of increased sexual desire in direct proportion to the amount of *Tribulus Terrestris* they were given.

- Other research has shown that cardiovascular health has been improved by *Tribulus Terrestris*; specifically it lowers cholesterol, the blood's triglyceride levels by almost 25% and glucose levels by almost 50%.

What is especially interesting is that all these benefits are attributed to the increase in testosterone levels that generally occurs when one takes *Tribulus Terrestris*.

How does it work?

Tribulus Terrestris works in two ways: by raising testosterone levels and increasing red blood cell counts (which help cardiovascular health, cholesterol and other blood related issues).

5. Non-Herbal Testosterone Deficiency and Libidinal Issue Remedies

These substances can greatly help the body although they are not herbal solutions to these problems. They do more than just increase your testosterone. They are also responsible for increased health throughout the body (within the blood vessels) and an enhanced libido. It is critical you work to find the balance that's right for you.

Enhancers

Enhancers should all be taken in 10x, 30x, or 100x strength tincture dosages.

Argentum Nitricum

What is it used for?

Erectile dysfunction.

Baryta Carbonica

What is it used for?

Treating impotence and libidinal issues.

Chaste Tree (Vitex angus castux)

What is it used for?

Treating erectile dysfunction, cognitive issues such as memory and focusing and the common cold.

Lycopodium

What is it used for?

Treating erectile dysfunction and improving confidence.

Testosterone Supplements

5% Variations of Testosterone Extract

Recommended daily dosage: 10x, 30x, and 100x strength tinctures

Oligometric ProanthyoCyanidins (OPC's)

Recommended daily dosage: 100 mg of grape seed extract and 100 mg resveratrol extract or 25 mg of red wine extract.

What are they used for?

OPC's are extracts that aid the blood in restoration and natural flow as well as absorption of antioxidants that can help with cognitive faculties and other health benefits.

Omega-3

Recommended daily dosage: 3,000 mg (3 grams).

What is it used for?

Omega-3 is a fatty acid used to break down fats within the blood vessels, preventing clots and reducing triglyceride levels.

Prelox (pycnogenol-L-Arginine)

Recommended daily dosage: 80 mg of pycnogenol and 3,000 mg (3 grams) of L-arginine

What is it used for?

Prelox is used to increase blood flow throughout the body and help with the processing of protein.

How does it work?

Prelox is a commercial product that actually contains two separate substances, pycnogenol and L-arginine. L-arginine is an amino acid that works to help the body in processing of protein. Pycnogenol has similar effects to aspirin but with added benefits to the efficiency of blood flow. These substances complement each other by enhancing the efficiency of blood flow AND increasing the level of nitric oxide.

Check out www.testosteroneboosterx.com, for total testosterone essential vitality.

Mineral Treatments

Zinc

Recommended daily dosage: 15 mg or ZMA.

What is it?

Dr. U. Mehta of the Indian Journal of Experimental Biology reported that diets low in the mineral zinc can actually result in the shrinking of the male sexual organ, lowered sperm counts and testosterone deficiencies.

Low levels of zinc are associated with damaging testosterone levels in the body. This is because zinc is key to the production of hormones related to sexual processes, including those that stimulate the prostate and produce sperm.

How does it work?

Zinc boosts testosterone production by stimulating the testes and testosterone receptors, allowing for more testosterone to flow throughout the body.

Zinc Monomethionine Aspartate (ZMA)

Recommended daily dosage: Vitamin B6 (11 mg) + Magnesium (450mg) + Zinc (30mg) -- 1 capsule per day.

What is it?

This is a combination of the minerals zinc, magnesium aspartate, and vitamin B6. A study published by the University of Washington on NCAA football players found that ZMA is significantly linked to increased muscle mass and testosterone levels.

How does it work?

It increases muscular strength and testosterone levels with the combined powers of the three minerals.

Section IV: How Your Diet Impacts Your Testosterone

How you eat impacts almost every aspect of your quality of life. Some foods can actually stimulate testosterone production naturally. But before we discuss how diet affects your testosterone levels, one very important point. This is ***not*** writing a diet book. Forget dieting; focus on eating *well*. That is my dietary advice to you. *Well* simply means a healthier, better you and is just a smarter route to go – not to mention that eating well is easier to maintain than following some rigid and crazy diet.

That's not to say that eating right has no health benefits. Eating right leads to a healthier body -- in terms of weight, in terms of health and in terms of testosterone. So let's start looking at ways you can benefit yourself by carefully selecting what you eat.

1. How You Should Be Eating

Eating healthy is much more than just what you do and don't put in your mouth. Eating is a set of habits. When do you eat? How much do you eat? What are your favorite foods? All of these factors come into play when considering if you're indulging in a healthy diet.

The truth is many people ignore this fact and suffer from terrible eating habits (like skipping breakfast -- sound familiar?). This section overviews healthy eating habits that will help you to reconsider how you eat and how that can impact your health and your levels of testosterone.

Eat less when you need less

When you arise in the morning you know what you'll be doing for the day so plan your diet accordingly. What I mean by this is you need to consider how much energy you will need and eat enough food to sustain you for your activities. Don't wait until you're starving to nosh on a bagel. If you know you're headed to the gym or doing strenuous activities, fill up at breakfast. The flip side: if all you'll be doing is playing video games perhaps you don't need an extra serving.

Eat more, but less

This somewhat teasing headline means that the best way to eat is to do so often, in smaller portions. The general rule of thumb is to eat every three hours that you intend to be up and working but to keep those meals small enough that you're not overloading yourself with calories.

Why does this work? Meals stimulate your body and initiate production of different chemical substances, like insulin. Insulin initiates fat building hormones. So, if you're trying to be healthier, and maybe shed those few extra pounds, consider eating more often – but less food!

Eat before you exercise

Working out takes a lot of energy and is a great time to burn fat. Ideally, one of the best times to eat should be shortly before you work out. A diet high in carbohydrates can help fuel your energy levels enough to even keep your workout going a little longer.

Smaller portions and bigger portions

Good big breakfasts

- Oatmeal
- Omelet
- Vegetables

There is a time and place for you to have both a big meal and a small meal but people usually eat them in the wrong order. People think they should start the day slow with a small meal but this is when you need your energy levels up – and have the most power to put that fuel to work. Conversely, evening is one of the worst times to have the bigger meal because you very rarely will be active enough to efficiently use the food.

Tip: If you eat a big meal in the morning and you're still hungry later – don't be afraid to snack! Fruits, yogurt, eggs and whole grains are very easy and quick snacks that can keep you going without filling you up unhealthily.

Habits aside, what you eat is just as important. It's not until you incorporate both good eating habits and eating healthy organic foods that you will see the results you want -- for your testosterone levels and your waistline.

2. What You Should Be Eating

All of the foods below will contribute in some way to rebuilding your testosterone storage and thus help you fight andropause (whether you're already in its clutches or trying to keep it from happening!).

Jettison the junk food

Foods to lose:

- White breads
- Pasta that isn't whole wheat
- Protein bars promising health benefits but high in sugars and genetically modified ingredients

Foods that are either nutritionally devoid or high in carbohydrates should be avoided in your efforts to eat well. This may seem common sense when it comes to things like potato chips but have you ever checked out the benefits of your white bread? Make sure you read the labels on your food carefully to determine whether they should be part of your daily meals.

Don't throw out all the foods that are high in fat

Exercise caution here. We're not saying bring back the brownies. But the truth is that some foods that are lower in fat have been associated with lowered levels of testosterone. The key is to strike an equilibrium.

You don't want fatty, nutritionally devoid foods as staples in your diet but you also don't want only low fat – you want the middle ground. (Think nuts, olive oil, certain animal fats, etc.). By adding foods that are *moderately* high in fat content you will be adding to your testosterone levels.

No we're not talking about TV dinners here. Look for canned goods that are actually, well, good for you. The key factors should be the sodium count and the sugar count (both of which should be low – the lower the better). Canned foods can be an excellent way to get a bit of variety in your diet without having to go to the market every day.

Nutrients you should look for

Niacin

Foods naturally high in niacin:

- Asparagus
- Bananas
- Broccoli
- Fish
- Lean meat
- Liver
- Peanuts
- Raw nuts
- Wheat Germ
- Whole Grains
- Yeast

Niacin is a great substance to include in your diet when suffering from testosterone deficiencies. It is a B-complex vitamin like riboflavin and thiamin, which all work together in concert. It has been linked to higher libido and ability to maintain erections.

Zinc

Foods naturally high in zinc:

- Caviar
- Chicken
- Duck
- Eggs
- Lamb
- Turkey
- Whole grains

We've already discussed the benefits of zinc supplements but it's worth noting that you can get a lot of zinc supplementation naturally through some of the foods above. More zinc, more testosterone.

Protein, protein, protein

Foods naturally high in protein:

- Cottage cheese
- Free-Range Eggs
- Certain types of fish like tuna, flounder and cod
- Free-Range Chicken
- Turkey (no skin)
- Lean red meat
- Grass-Fed Beef
- Quinoa

NOTE: Avoid designer "protein shakes" or bars. Although they are high in 'protein,' it is synthetic and often laced with extra estrogen – something your body does not need and will not help your testosterone!

Protein, the ancient Greek word for "primary nutrient," is an essential part of any diet and should regularly be included in most of your meals. Protein is important because it is a prerequisite that triggers the production of hormones associated with growth processes (like muscle building, insulin regulation, etc.) as well as strengthening the thyroid. This means protein helps your body to increase testosterone, decrease fat and regulate itself better.

How much you should have? 0.84 - 1 gram per pound. So if you weigh 200 pounds, you should be eating between 168 - 200 grams of protein daily.

Organic Vegetables

Good-for-testosterone-vegetables

- Beans
- Bell peppers
- Broccoli
- Brussels sprouts
- Cabbage
- Collard Greens
- Kale
- Lentils
- Spinach
- Zucchini

Vegetables are chock full of minerals, fiber, phytochemicals and antioxidants. All of these substances are fantastic for you -- not just for your testosterone levels but to prepare you for physical activity. They raise your energy levels, your ability to focus and yes, your libido. Mix in some veggies with that meal!

That being said, you need to STEAM these vegetables in most cases (5 - 10 minutes is ideal) at 212 degrees. Steaming vegetables is a thyroid protective action. Some raw vegetables contain ingredients that can inhibit the thyroid (and counteract certain medications).

Variety

Variety isn't just the spice of life; it's also the best way to get a healthy body. Don't just focus on proteins or vegetables. Mix it up from time to time to ensure you have a healthy *and well rounded* eating regimen. Eat your grains but also your berries. Remember your old favorites but never be afraid to seek out new ones. This not only keeps you healthier, it also makes it easier to spice up your diet by trying different kinds of meals. This also decreases your chances of getting bored with healthy eating and quitting.

3. Eating Right

Eating right doesn't just mean a higher level of testosterone -- it also means a healthier you overall. Eating right translates to more energy, more muscle, more desire to do the things that you love, less unhealthy weight gain and absolutely a healthier level of testosterone and libidinal energy overall.

4. Keep Hydrated!

Some people work really hard to eat right, and eat with great habits, but forget their body's need to stay hydrated. Water is one of the best gifts you can give your body and one of the worst punishments you can inflict when you deprive yourself of hydration.

If you aren't drinking your daily amount of water (64 ounces, or 8 oz. of eight full glasses), your kidneys suffer. They are your waste disposal organs – you want them performing at peak levels. If kidneys function at a diminished level, they impose extra work on other organs (like the liver). This also inefficiently uses the fuels you have worked so hard to accumulate. So you see, failing to drink enough fluids can be just as detrimental to a diet as having an hourly doughnut.

Additionally, because hydration affects how your body uses its resources, it is especially critical that you are hydrated if you're planning on intense physical activity. Budd Coates, a fitness consultant for 'Men's Health' magazine, has been quoted as saying you should ALWAYS have a bottle of water within arm's reach when you're planning to exercise.

Interestingly, research on the subject has actually found that often when we think we're hungry, we're actually thirsty. So the next time you feel a bit peakish (but you know you've already eaten), go get a glass of cold water.

Does the kind of water I drink matter?

The short answer is yes. Nowadays there are different 'kinds' of water, all claiming to be the best for you. Research reveals the characteristics of water you want. Consult the following list (rated from highest to lowest quality) when considering water.

1) Deionized
2) Filtered
3) Spring
4) Tap (or from plastic bottles)

Drink up and drink often!

5. Summary

By paying attention to what you're eating, how you're eating and when you're drinking, you will be well on your way to becoming a better you – even before the supplements kick in. That gut you've been trying to lose for so long won't be so hard to get rid of. Your arms may bulk up a little more. Your energy levels will have you convinced you’re sleeping 12 hours per night instead of 8.

You will be repaid for every bit of effort you invest in your nutritional intake and your testosterone levels will thank you too.

Section V: Sex, the Ultimate Testosterone Boost

The health benefits of sex:

- Sex triggers the release of endorphins – a hormone associated with increased mood and *painkilling!* Some researchers, such as Beverly Whipple, Ph.D. even believe that sex can increase your tolerance for pain!

- Sex works out your entire respiratory system with your 'heavy' (deep) breathing

- Sex lowers cholesterol

- Sex stimulates weight loss!

- Orgasms help your body in numerous ways, from stimulating pleasurable feelings and testosterone production to clearing out your glands by flushing fluid through them.

Hopefully this won't come as too much of a surprise to you but sex is an extremely physical activity. When you have sex you engage multiple areas of your body in (rampant) physical activity, and physical activity isn't bad for you at all – especially not your testosterone levels. We'll discuss the importance of exercise a bit later in the book but for now, let's talk about sex.

In terms of holding different positions and stretching different ways, there are some exercises that can help you train your body to be better at sex. Flexibility is key. Let's look at the exercises by the body parts that are affected most.

1. Abdomen

Strengthening your abdomen vastly improves your sexual ability. Your entire body relies on the strength of your abdomen when you're making love. The best way to strengthen your abdomen is by using exercises that target that part of the body the most -- crunches.

To perform a crunch you need to lay back, holding your body straight (you can tell you're straight when your lower back is flat against the floor and your neck is relaxed). Ensure that your feet are completely flat on the floor. Now, keeping your back on the floor and neck completely relaxed, pull your torso up toward your knees, holding yourself a few inches off from the ground for a moment at a time.

How much should you crunch? When you begin crunches you will need to start slow -- three sets of ten should be a good beginning. The easier the crunches become over time, the more of them you should do. Work your way up to doing 3 sets of 20 repetitions each.

2. Hips and Groin

When it comes to your hips, the name of the game is flexibility. You need to be able to move not just back and forth, but from side to side. The best way to improve your flexibility is through stretching so we'll review some stretches to help your pelvis develop floor strength.

Butterfly Stretch

Lay on the bed with your legs bent and feet once again flat. Use your hands to turn your feet so that they are flat against each other (knees bent to the side). Slowly exhale and allow your knees to tug themselves toward the bed.

How much should you butterfly? Hold it for 10 seconds as strong as you can and then relax.

Penis Exercises

Okay, so there's no Bowflex for this part of your body. But you can work out your love muscle and do so in a way that will result in better orgasms. Ready? Here we go.

Sit on the edge of a bed or couch. Arouse yourself. Feel the muscle that moves your penis (either up and down or side to side) and flex those muscles. Flexing increases blood flow. And more blood flow means a harder erection.

3. Why Do This?

So why should you bother exercising for the sake of lovemaking? Two reasons:

1) You will become a better lover. (Never a bad goal).
2) Orgasms stimulate testosterone production!!!

Orgasms are a natural (and really fun) way to get your body not only into shape – sex makes great exercise – but also to stimulate the production of testosterone. And consider this: even if you don't think you're having sex "that often," if you orgasm just three times per week you burn up to 7,500 calories. It's the equivalent of running 75 miles!

Sex is a great way to work off a hard day and still get a workout, *and* it helps to naturally boost your testosterone. So whether you're on your own or with a partner, don't be afraid to indulge!

Section VI: Weight Loss, the Testosterone Solution

Often when you're targeting one area of your life for improvement -- testosterone levels in this case -- you start thinking about other areas in your health that could use some attention. For example, that abdomen you used to be able to see.

Don't feel bad. We've all lost the washboard at one time or another but the truth is, you can get it back. I will not mention diets because I don't put a lot of stock in them. However, this guide has already offered advice on how to eat well and eat right (which should already be helping). So we'll give some simple advice on how to lose that gut.

Step 1) Stimulate your metabolism. Set the stage for weight loss by adding foods high in metabolism stimulation, fat burning and low in glycemic carbohydrates.

Step 2) Take out the empty carbs (high glycemic carbohydrates, listed below) *from your diet*. All they do is fill your body with insulin it doesn't need (which is then converted to fat).

Step 3) Engage your body in physical activity, preferably with strength exercises. Strength training will ensure that your body is physically engaged and working to build muscle. If you're looking to lose weight, why not kill two birds with one stone and convert that fatty tissue to muscular tissue? Strength training should be taken up to three times a week for maximum effectiveness.

Step 4) Supplement your diet as necessary. Again, don't think just pills. Eat vegetables (and other organic foods) high in antioxidants, vitamins and minerals. It will stimulate your fat burning bodily substances.

Following these tips is a start, but ideally you also need to recognize your ideal calorie count when it comes to your daily meals. This takes a bit more of understanding of the different food groups, so this chapter gives you an overview.

1. Foods high in glycemic carbohydrates

We've already mentioned that high glycemic carbohydrates are bad for your body but what kinds of foods are they? Let's look at some of the high glycemic foods from different food groups to give you a better idea of how to spot them. Once you know how to identify them, avoid them where possible or at least until you achieve your initial weight loss goals.

Know that glycemic foods fight against your body's ability to lose weight. After you've shed those pounds it shouldn't be as much of an issue. For now, try to avoid them. When in doubt about a food, read the label.

Starches

- Bagels, breads (read the label if in doubt)
- Bakery type products (cakes, cookies, doughnuts, pies)
- Cereals with more than 5 grams per serving
- Millet
- "Starchy" Veggies (potatoes, corn, peas, butternut and acorn squash)
- Waffles
- White bread
- White rice

Sugars

Maximum intake should be set to 15 - 18 grams per day

- All juices except vegetable juice
- Candy
- Dairy (sweetened milks, cow's milk)
- Fruits (fresh and dried)

After reading this list, you may be wondering what you'll be able to have on this weight loss journey. The following is a list of foods that are lower in glycemic carbs.

2. Foods low in glycemic carbohydrates

Complex Carbohydrates

75 - 100 grams daily

- Amaranth
- Barley
- Brown rice (Orzo)
- Buckwheat
- Legumes (black beans, garbanzo beans, lentils, red and white kidney beans)
  1/2 cup to 3/4 cup maximum.
- Nuts
  Avoid peanuts as they inhibit the thyroid
- Oatmeal
- Rye bread
- "Non-Starchy" Veggies (eggplant, kale, pumpkin, red peppers, tomatoes, summer squash, zucchini)
- Whole grain pasta
  1 cooked cup 3 days/week
- Whole wheat bagels
- Quinoa

Fats

100 calories, 10 - 15 grams per serving, 2 - 4 daily servings

- Avocado
- Coconut oil
- Flaxseed oil
- Mixed nuts (without peanuts)
- Olive oil

Proteins

0.5 - 0.75 grams * pound of your goal weight (example 180 lbs. * .5 - .75 = 90 - 135 grams daily)

- Beef
  6 - 8 ounces 3 - 4 times per week
- Chicken (leaner the better, no skin)
- Dairy (cottage, cheddar, Swiss, Monterey cheeses)
- Eggs
  1 - 2 daily per week if you want
- Fish (particularly those high in Omega-3 fatty acids)
- Ham
- Pork
- Protein Powders (egg, milk or whey types)
  Should have no more than 2 - 3 grams of sugar per serving
- Turkey

Sugars

Again, limit is 15 - 18 grams daily until fitness goals achieved

- Fruits low in sugar (apricots, blackberries, blueberries, huckleberry, plums, raspberries, strawberries)
- Vegetable juice (no more than 6 - 7 grams per serving)
- Sugar free items

3. Free Foods

These foods require no limitation. Have as much as you want!

- All spices
- Celery
- Chives
- Lemon juice
- Mushrooms
- Parsley
- Stevia
- Tea
- Unsweetened or Stevia sweetened gelatin
- Unsweetened almond milk

4. Supplements That Can Help

If you're really looking to improve not just your weight but your physique, you definitely need to consider your nutrition (which we've already discussed at length). It's also critical that you examine supplements.

Check out www.testosteroneboosterx.com, for total testosterone essential vitality.

The following is information taken from Dr. Karlis Ullis' book 'Super T' for specifically testosterone targeting supplements. We have updated the information as research has evolved, and feel that these items should be taken in supplement form.

Note that one supplement could contain multiple parts so keep an eye open for a multi-vitamin/supplement.

Antioxidants

Antioxidants are linked to improved cognitive abilities, anti-aging effects, the prevention of free radical cells (which can lead to cancer) and have the ability to help combat the effects of numerous other illnesses.

- Alpha and beta carotenes daily dosage – 5 - 20 mg
- Flavonoid mixtures:
  Grape seed extract daily dosages – 50 - 300 mg
  Green tea extract daily dosage – 150 mg (1 - 3 daily)
- Minerals (Copper chealte – 1 - 3 mg; Manganese – 5 - 15 mg; Selenium – 100 - 500mg; Zinc – 15 - 55mg)
- Resveratrol daily dosage – 100 - 200 mg
- Quercetin daily dosage – 500 - 1,000 mg
- Vitamin A daily dosage – 5000 IU
- Vitamin C daily dosage – 500 - 1,000 mg
- Vitamin D3 daily dosage – 1,000 - 2,000 IU
- Vitamin E daily dosages – 400 - 1,000 IU

B Vitamins

B Vitamins helps prevent cancer, depression, heart disease, immune system problems memory preservation and senility.

- B1 (thiamine) daily dosage – 50,100 mg (1 - 2 times)
- B2 (riboflavin) daily dosage – 10-20 mg (1 - 2 times)
- B3 (niacinamide) daily dosage – 20-200 mg (1 - 2 times)
- B5 (pantothenate) daily dosage – 250 mg (1 - 2 times)
- B6 (pyridoxine) daily dosage – 25-50 mg (1 - 2 times)
- B12 (sublingual methyl cobalamin) daily dosage – 500 mcg (1 - 2 times)
- Folic acid (take with B12) daily dosage – 400-500 mcg (1-2 times)

Herbs/Spices

These products often have curative and flavorful powers, so don't take them lightly. They can be taken as desired.

- Cayenne, black pepper, turmeric, fresh parsley
- Garlic daily dosage – 1 - 2 cloves (4 grams; 2 - 3 times per day)
  If taken in supplements: 1 - 2 capsules containing 10 mg allicin or 4,000 mcg total allicin potential (2 - 3 times daily, after eating)
- Gingko Biloba daily dosage – 40 - 80 mg (1-3 times per day)

Macrominerals

- Calcium chelate daily dosage – 200 - 600 mg
- Magnesium chelate daily dosage – 250 - 800mg

Mitochondrial Protectors

- Alpha-Lipoic acid daily dosage – 50 - 600 mg
- CoQ10 (ubiqunone type)
- N-acetyl L-carnitine – 100 - 2,000 mg
- N-acetyl Cysteine – 100 - 1,200 mg

Miscellaneous

These should be included with your daily vitamin and mineral list with the exceptions of betaine HCL which can be found in its own supplement class at your local food store.

- Betaine HCL daily dosage – 100 - 150 mg
- Vitamin K (phytonadione) daily dosage – 60 - 300 mcg
- Biotin daily dosage – 100 - 300 mcg
- Boron daily dosage – 1 - 6 mg
- Choline daily dosage – 50 - 500 mg
- Iodine daily dosage – 50 - 100 mcg
- Inositol daily dosage – 30 - 100 mg
- Potassium daily dosage – 200 - 500 mg
- 7-Keto DHEA daily dosage – 100 mg a day

Oils

- Cod liver oil daily dosage – 1 tbsp.
- Flaxseed oil daily dosage – 1 - 2 tbsp.
- Olive oil – 1 - 2 tbsp.

Trace Minerals

- Chromium (polynicotinate) daily dosage -- 200 - 400 mcg
- Molybdenum (trioxide or sodium molybate) daily dosage – 50 - 600 mcg

5. Problems Related to Obesity

Obesity has reached nearly pandemic levels in North America. There's much we haven't understood over the years but research is constantly working to expand our knowledge. One of the most recent discoveries is that obesity has the effects of a disease. When you are obese your body produces inflammatory cytokines (something that non-obese people do not produce), causing a host of problems.

Inflammatory cytokines leads to heart problems, arthritis, testosterone issues, weight gain and increases of estrogen -- a big problem for any self-respecting man. Another issue with obesity and testosterone is that people who are obese actually convert their testosterone stores to estrogen. This not only causes plenty of medical problems but makes it difficult to just maintain one's masculinity. These facts are not here to scare you but rather to encourage you to consider a weight loss program if you are currently struggling with obesity.

Taking supplements and following nutritional guides is only a part of a weight loss strategy. The final piece to the puzzle is finding your ideal amount of calories and limiting yourself to that quantity. This will prevent buildup of unnecessary fat within your body.

Calories are simply components of heat that the body uses whenever it needs energy. When you have extra calories that remain unused, they are stored as fat. The amount of calories that you need depends largely on your individual energy expenditures, your base metabolic rate and your level of physical activity.

So let's do some calculating.

Step 1) Your basal metabolic rate, BMR, is the rate that your metabolism functions at. If you are in a weight loss program, your BMR is probably currently low (if it were high you wouldn't have anything to burn off). Let's assume a typical sedentary BMR rate of 10.

Step 2) Your weight. Weigh yourself on a scale and record your current weight as well as your desired weight loss goal. Let's assume a body weight of 200 lbs.

Step 3) Multiply your current weight by your BMR. 200 X 10 = 2,000 in our current example. This is the daily calorie intake that would be necessary to maintain your current body weight.

Step 4) Now, since we know we don't want to maintain our current body weight, figure out what you want to weigh. In our example we will use 175. Now multiply 175 by your BMR (10 in this case) to get 1,750 calories.

As you may have guessed, this indicates the calorie intake to maintain that weight – and thus will function as your caloric limit to reach that weight.

NOTE: Losing too many calories at once is unhealthy – be realistic. This is your best shot at a long term level of success.

Step 5) Function with that limit as your daily limit.

6. How to Keep to a Calorie Limit

Now that you have a calorie limit you may be intimidated, worrying about every little thing you eat. But remember, there are ways to eat healthier that will naturally bring this count down.

The following are eating habit help tips to enable you to cut down your calorie intake.

Eat often, but less

This is the same tip from above, but a little more specific. When trying to lose weight, eat 6 small meals per day: Breakfast, brunch, lunch, snack, dinner and snack. This is how a three hour meal schedule actually works.

Don't skip meals!

Cut down on sugar

If you can eliminate sugar your body will thank you. If you don't want to completely eliminate sugar, at least limit your intake to strictly 15 - 18 grams per day. This will stop sugar from interfering with your weight loss goals and enable you to reach the target weight you want.

Read labels

Reading labels is just good sense; you know exactly what you put into your body and what your body gets in return. This will help you meet your goals in no time.

Watch your portion sizes

You can use food labels, measuring cups or a food scale -- just know how much food you putting into your body.

Keep track of what you're eating on paper

Writing down what you eat has two purposes. 1) It keeps you accountable and 2) it allows you to see your weaknesses on paper. Where did you eat more or less than you should? Why?

Meal requirements

Every meal should include:

- 1 - 2 tbsp. of healthy fats
- 15 - 20 grams of protein
- 20 - 25 grams of carbohydrates

This should provide you with a balanced meal. Excessive indulgence in these substances results in more weight; moderation results in weight loss. The decision is yours.

Creating Your Menu

Now you're ready to make a plan. Let's look at some tips before you create a menu. I will include one of mine as an example, along with a sample food diary. However, you need to find what works best for you individually.

Perhaps you prefer to keep track of your meals at the end of the day or maybe you want to swap fish with turkey. Whatever the case, consider the following tips when planning what to eat.

- Keep writing down what you're eating. This helps you to stay accountable to your calorie limit. It also provides you a reference when you think, "I really liked what I ate on ... day...what was that again?"

- Keep your calorie limit in mind! Calculate it and abide by it. Remember, you're aiming for better memory, better health and a more lively sex life. Are a few doughnuts really worth the sacrifice?

- Use the lists provided for advice on "good" and "bad" foods. Mix and match, find recipes with multiple good ingredients and experiment!

Below you will find a sample menu and sample food diary to get you started. Print them out, make copies for yourself and tailor it if you like! Own your weight loss -- this is your journey.

Sample Menus

Breakfast:

4 ounces of fish (pickled herring perhaps), One ½ of a whole wheat bagel, ½ cup berries, coffee or tea, black or with half-half cream and Stevia sweetener.

Snack:

2 hard-boiled eggs or 1 - 2 ounces of cheese with 4 whole wheat crackers, ½ avocado with 1 Tbsp. olive oil and Cajun seasoning.

Lunch:

1 cup cottage cheese with ½ cup fresh or water packed pineapple, 1 slice low-carb bread with 2 Tbsp. hummus.

Or

1 can water packed tuna with 2 Tbsp. olive oil mayo, 2 slices low carb bread or Flat-out or 8" round.

Snack:

1 oz. of unsalted mixed nuts (no peanuts), 1 plum, white tea with Stevia.

Dinner:

6 - 8 ounces of baked, spiced chicken or 4 - 6 ounces broiled grass fed beef, ½ cup steamed brown rice, ½ cup baked summer squash, 4 ounces of asparagus with stir-fried red peppers.

Dessert:

1 cup berries with real whipped cream.

Snack:

4 ounces turkey with 1 Tbsp. olive oil mayonnaise or ¼ cup unsalted mixed nuts (no peanuts) or 2 Tbsp. almond/cashew/sunflower seed butter with green apple slices.

Sample Food Tracking Page

You can arrange a sheet however you want to record your intake, but you must abide by the following rules: Keep track of your 1) calorie intake, 2) protein intake, 3) carbohydrate and 4) sugar intake. Stick to your limitations and recommendations for best results!

Breakfast	Calories	Protein	Carbs	Sugar
Lunch	Calories	Protein	Carbs	Sugar
Dinner	Calories	Protein	Carbs	Sugar
Snacks	Calories	Protein	Carbs	Sugar

Section VII: The Importance of Physical Activity

This shouldn't much of a surprise but when it comes to being healthy, physical activity is something of a requirement. Physical activity helps your body to stimulate the production of a variety of hormones that are great for fat burning, testosterone building and overall health.

1. Benefits of Exercising

- Exercise helps you to increase your strength, flexibility and overall happiness
- Physical activity has been linked to a reduced risk of hypertension, heart attack, depression and diabetes
- Regular exercise helps sleep regulation
- Physical exercise helps you to construct your physique by building muscle slowly but surely

Want to know another reason you should be happy to work out? You're going to like this. Try working out with your partner. Want to know why? Exercise releases endorphins -- feel good hormones -- and creates the desire to be physically active. A workout can be a very arousing time for a couple with great sex afterward.

Many men may think this only works for the young guy with the 6 pack abs when he's running around shirtless. Not so -- exercise promotes sexual behavior due to the release of a combination of endorphins and the release of testosterone. Remember, testosterone is directly linked to sexual desire. She doesn't need you to look like Studly Beefcakes, she needs you to look like a man – and you can certainly do something about that!

"Any form of physical activity is going to raise your levels of testosterone" Clinical psychologist Karen Donahey, Ph.D.

2. Types of Physical Activity

But what type of physical activity should you be doing? There are three primary areas you need to target in your physical activity:

- Strength (to ensure you have the muscles instead of just flab as you lose fat)
- Flexibility
- Cardiovascular – This refers to your entire respiratory system, specifically your heart and your lungs.

This chapter will overview exercises for each of these areas to ensure you are getting the maximal health and testosterone benefits. You'll be in the pink in no time!

NOTE: If you are concerned that you may be unable to do a certain type of exercise, don't force it initially. Seek professional medical advice before starting a new routine if you fear injury.

Your Strength

Exercises that increase your strength and your flexibility often go hand in hand with the following exercises.

Names of the muscles (so you can know what you're working out)

- Latissimus dorsi, deltoids, triceps, pectoral muscles AND rhomboids (upper body muscles)
- Quadriceps (thigh muscles)
- Gluteus complex (Hips and behind muscle groups).

Exercises to Work Out With:

Each of these can be worked with in sets of 10 at a time. Try to get up to 3 done.

Knee bends – Stand with your legs shoulder width apart. Check to see that your feet are pointed straight in front of you and slowly exhale as you lower your body into a squatting position. Hold for a moment and straight yourself back up while inhaling.

Pushups – Lay on the floor on your stomach. Position yourself so that you are resting your weight on your feet (toes specifically) and your hands (shoulder width apart, directly beneath yourself). Lift your body upwards, holding it as straight as you can and exhale. Hold for a moment then release, inhaling as you lower yourself. Repeat.

Alternate pushups – Do the normal push up, except have your knees hold you up (instead of your toes).

Weights – If you're looking for a challenge, try doing a squat with weights attached to either your legs or arms. This is not necessarily a necessity but can help to build muscle and keep your work out varied, which is extremely important. Just keep in mind you don't want to overdo it, so work with weights that are only moderately difficult to lift (rather than extremely) to prevent strain.

Your Flexibility

Although many strengthening exercises are also flexibility exercises, there are separate exercises that you can do specifically to increase your flexibility. Have you ever heard the saying “use it or lose it”? It directly applies here. We lose flexibility as we age, and the way to counteract it is exercise. So the good news? You CAN counteract these effects.

Quadriceps

Lay down on your side and pull both of your knees slowly up toward your chest. Pull your heel toward your behind until you feel the stretch. Hold that for a few seconds and repeat it ten times. Then switch legs.

Trunk stretch

Side reaching – Stand up straight, placing two hands behind your head while leaning to the right as much as you can. Hold it for a few seconds, release and do ten repetitions before switching sides.

Leg bending – Sit on the floor with your knees pointed to opposite walls (bent at 90 degrees). Contract the muscles in your upper body as you lean towards the knees.

Reverse trunk stretch

Lay down on your back, keeping one leg flat and the other bent. Pull your bent knee toward your opposite shoulder, hold it and release. Do 10 repetitions.

Hamstrings

General – Stand with your legs shoulder width apart. Take one foot and extend it while bending the opposite leg to keep yourself stable. Flex your extended foot to really feel the stretch but keep your weight focused on your body itself. Do ten reps.

Straight leg – Lay on your back, bending one knee at a time. Pull your body upwards toward your knee that is not bent and hold for a few seconds. Do 10 repetitions and switch your legs.

Calf stretches

Stand with your feet shoulder width apart. Step forward with one leg, shifting your weight onto that leg and resting your hand on the opposite leg for stability. Do ten repetitions and switch legs.

Pelvic tilts

Lay down on your back. Lift your right thigh and pull it towards the chest, bending the knee. Hold for a few seconds then release, letting your leg naturally return to its position. Complete ten repetitions and then switch legs (doing ten repetitions again).

Pelvic tilt alternative

Begin in the same starting position, slowly pulling both knees to your chest this time. You can do just ten reps when you do both legs at once.

3. The Cardiovascular System

People may suggest you start running or take up jogging but we won't do that. Why not? Running is more often than not done improperly and can often lead to injury in your joints, along the heels and even in your shins.

The same goes for the suggestion of weight lifting and other popular exercises. These exercises also do not differentiate between burning muscle and burning fat so they are not helpful in forming a physique or boosting your testosterone. Truth is, in some cases the wrong exercises actually result in lower levels of testosterone – the opposite of your goal here.

What Do We Recommend?

- Bicycling – Phenomenal for your cardiovascular system AND your strength – and you can do it in the gym or outside!

- StairMaster – This is what experts refer to as a "low impact aerobic aid." Low impact aerobics are great, the risk for hurting yourself is minimized and you can still really tone your body and get your system working for you.

- Swimming – It's really hard to hurt yourself when you're in the water and it's a great place to work out. The joints especially are very easily exercised but will not endure long term damage in water. That's why swimming is one of our favorites.

These exercises each work to give your whole system a workout and do so in a way that minimizes your risk of damage. You can do any or all of these exercises but try to pick at least one. Perform exercising in one to two minute jaunts at your chosen exercise then take a break. Repeat until you've worked out 20 - 30 minutes. These cycles should be increased by five minutes at a time as your resistance increases for them to continue to have an impact.

If you'd like, you can vary the exercises you do (i.e., StairMaster today, swim tomorrow) to keep your interest up and your body challenged! Just remember to be safe.

4. Safety tips for working out the cardiovascular system:

- Don't use sports to get yourself fit. Get fit and then play sports. Otherwise you risk injury and damage from running improperly, etc.
- Don't indulge in aerobics and weight lifting simultaneously (EVER)
- Do not do more than 45 minutes of aerobic exercise in a single exercise session or in a single day

5. Change It Up – Progression and How It Should Effect Your Workout

If you were learning how to juggle, and you had figured how to throw one ball with one hand and catch it in the other, would you count yourself a master juggler? No, you'd likely aim to where you could juggle three or maybe even five balls before you'd consider yourself an expert.

So why would you expect that your workout should stay the same even after you begin to improve? Answer -- you shouldn't expect this. As you progress in your abilities you need to advance your workout.

This doesn't mean you need to aim for 25 hours of cycling per week some day. It just means if you did three hours this week, you could consider doing five next week. And if you don't want to do six the next week, perhaps you should try doing three hours cycling and two hours with a StairMaster.

The goal is to consistently keep your body challenged so you can continue to grow and not get stuck in the rut of having improved a little bit... and so now your body is conditioned to a certain point and that's as far as it goes.

A warning: you are not out to hurt yourself. If you experience pain after working out, it's okay but don't continue working out the same way the very next day. Give yourself a break. Allow your body to restore itself.

Another thing you should understand about exercising -- you aren't building muscle when you're working out. You're building muscle when you're eating right and doing other things that stimulate your body's production of hormones that lead to growth of muscle mass.

Section VIII: When Will You See Results?

I constantly come across doctors who treat numerous patients who could benefit from this treatment. However, these doctors are convinced their patients' symptoms are just a normal part of aging. Apparently some men accept the idea that weight gain, crankiness, lack of motivation and indeed reduction in sex drive are just all part and parcel of making your way through the world. By starting testosterone therapy you are acknowledging you are one of those who know otherwise.

That said, this journey can take a lot of dedication and research so at this point you may wonder about results. I would like to encourage you with the story of my friend Chris.

Chris is a gentleman I first encountered at an anti-aging conference. He is physically active, fun spirited, vital and healthy, brilliant... and 83 years old. I once teased Chris by saying he must have found the Fountain of Youth on one of his many trips, but he responded quite seriously. You see, Chris is all of the things I mentioned but he is also extremely health conscious. He didn't just take vitamins or just exercise or just eat well... he did all those things. And while they worked for a while they were not enough until he added testosterone therapy to his life.

The vitamins, the exercise -- all of it really did help Chris remain very healthy well into his 60s but when he hit 70 he started to experience changes. He was exhausted all the time, he started gaining weight and all of a sudden sex didn't seem all that important any more. Sound familiar? Well, Chris wasn't ready to throw in the towel. He had been active all of his life. Moping around watching TV all day was not an option. So he went to see his doctor.

The doctor only had to run a few tests before he found that, you guessed it, Chris's testosterone levels were low. Chris became slightly hopeful; this was something he may be able to target.

As it happened, one of his friends had told him about testosterone enhancements before -- specifically ginseng, Maca and Tribulus Terrestris supplements. When Chris heard he was suffering from a testosterone deficiency he knew this was something he wanted to try.

Within three months, Chris found the supplements had made a dramatic difference. At four months, Chris felt as though the drop in energy never happened! Now, you'd never know he struggled at all except when he so openly sits before you, sharing his story.

Chris is a living testament to the power of testosterone supplements and dedication. He refused to accept decline as a normal part of aging. He did not take any reduction in sex drive lying down and when he worked to try those supplements, he was rewarded. When people ask me if it's "too late" or if they can recover from the damage done, I point out Chris.

You may think that three to four months sounds manageable for the kind of results he got, and it is, but actually it does not always take that long. The following chapter overviews a six week guide to what you should expect to see on your testosterone supplement journey, and yes, there will be changes within that time! By emphasizing what to look for, you'll notice in detail as the symptoms disappear.

Six Week Guide to the Signs of Testosterone Recovery

Everyone has their own schedule when it comes to testosterone recovery levels. This timeline is a guide for the disappearance of symptoms in the average patient. Most people's results tend to follow this timeline. If your results don't, stay calm. Just be aware for when these things do happen for you.

Week 1: The Depression Is Over and It's Time For Some Fun!

Say goodbye to feelings of depression and hello to that new desire to maintain an erection. This is the beginning -- a wonderful time when your body is first astounded by the induction of extra testosterone. These feelings typically take effect between two to four days after you begin your regimen.

You'll be encouraged as these effects take charge, which will only serve to lift your mood. Things seem a little less stressful. Your confidence begins to grow. And you seem to have all this energy for those projects you've been neglecting around the house. Enjoy this feeling and this time -- it's here to stay!

It should be noted that testosterone supplementation is not an anti-depressant and those medications should not be replaced by testosterone supplements.

Week 2: Go For A Run -- It Won't Hurt!

Okay, it doesn't have to be a run. It can be any kind of an urge for physical activity but chances are by now you'll be craving it. And if you indulge this craving you'll be rewarded, as you start to feel your strength returning.

The really wonderful thing? It's not going to 'hurt' your joints because testosterone's anti-inflammatory properties will likely have taken effect by then, relieving many familiar pains.

Week 3: Continued Strength and Muscular Gain, and Dramatic Weight Loss

If you've been working out at this point, you'll notice by now that you can go as long as you once did! Testosterone helps push you into longer workouts without the typical lingering aches and pain that once followed your exercise.

That said, you should be careful. Feeling strong like this can cause you to overextend yourself. Exercise caution or you'll seriously hurt yourself by pushing too hard. A healthy amount of exertion is fine -- just don't do it too hard.

1 pound of weight lost = 1 pound of muscle gained

Another benefit to working out, if indeed you have been, is by now your body should be feeling the effects. This means increased tone and muscular formation and eventually weight loss if you keep at it.

Week 4 - 5: Increased Focus

Here is where the benefits to your mind start to take effect. When your testosterone levels are sufficiently high, your mind stays sharp and allows you to focus far easier and more efficiently. This manifests itself in memory recovery and a general feeling of mental acuity.

Week 6: Enjoying All of the Effects

This is where all of the effects come together. By week six you'll notice a significant improvement resulting from your testosterone therapy. You'll feel genuinely better and people will note the changes in your appearance. You'll possess a confidence you haven't felt since you were in your 20s.

Congratulations -- you are a man and a wholly developed one at that! In less than two months, you've recovered from a testosterone deficiency.

Conclusions

You've done it -- you've reached the end! We've provided you with a lot of information, tips and advice. We've offered you knowledge and help, and all for one goal: to increase your levels of testosterone.

The great news? This can be done!

Many men with low testosterone have seen their levels increase by following this system. A summary of what this program entails:

- Monitor your testosterone levels
  Are you deficient? How long has this gone on? How are you progressing as you go through this program?

- Eat well
  Eat right, adjust your eating habits and continue to eat smart.

- Become physically active

- Look into supplements for anything you're missing

Whether you're just starting to notice a lack of energy or suffered from a lack of sexual desire for the past five years, there is help available. Feel free to reread chapters as needed and take notes on the issues that trouble you. Print these sheets for tracking your eating habits.

Most of all? Good luck! You are on the road to a better you, both health wise and testosterone wise.

Please note that the guidance provided in this book is not meant to act as a substitute for medical advice. If you are concerned about an area of your life, be it a lack of sex drive, weight gain and especially a lack of happiness, seek medical attention!

IF a health professional finds a testosterone deficiency, this book can more than help but don't just self-diagnose and then move from there.

Remember, this guide focuses on natural solutions. When you work with natural methods, you dramatically lower the risk of harming yourself from unintended side effects.

If you found this book helpful, please share a couple of sentences and a 4-5 star review on Amazon. It would mean a great deal to me.

If you have any questions or comments, feel free to email me at nick@mensgrowth.com, I try to reply to all questions that come in and that I am able to.

Resources

Learn More

Visit MensGrowth.com to check out the latest advice for men who look to be ambitious... master their lifestyle... perform in the bedroom... experience better health, wealth and personal growth...

www.MensGrowth.com

Newsletter

Click here to stay connected to our MensGrowth.com newsletter for strategies on better health, increased wealth, style, sex and personal growth news sent right to your inbox.

www.MensGrowth.com/join

Recommended Resources

Check out www.testosteroneboosterx.com, for total testosterone essential vitality.

Made in the USA
Middletown, DE
27 October 2022